CAMBRIDGE PUBLIC HEALTH SERIES

UNDER THE EDITORSHIP OF

G. S. Graham-Smith, M.D., and J. E. Purvis, M.A.

University Lecturer in Hygiene and Secretary to the Sub-Syndicate for Tropical Medicine

University Lecturer in Chemistry and Physics in their application to Hygiene and Preventive Medicine, and Secretary to the State Medicine Syndicate

T0372348

OCCUPATIONS

OCCUPATIONS

FROM THE SOCIAL, HYGIENIC AND MEDICAL POINTS OF VIEW

BY

SIR THOMAS OLIVER, M.A., M.D. LL.D., D.Sc., F.R.C.P.

Professor of the Principles and Practice of Medicine, University of Durham
and Hon. Consulting Physician to the Royal Victoria Infirmary
Newcastle-upon-Tyne

Cambridge:

at the University Press

1916

CAMBRIDGE
UNIVERSITY PRESS

University Printing House, Cambridge CB2 8BS, United Kingdom

Published in the United States of America by Cambridge University Press, New York

Cambridge University Press is part of the University of Cambridge.

It furthers the University's mission by disseminating knowledge in the pursuit of
education, learning and research at the highest international levels of excellence.

www.cambridge.org
Information on this title: www.cambridge.org/9781107419216

© Cambridge University Press 1916

First published 1916
First paperback edition 2014

A catalogue record for this publication is available from the British Library

ISBN 978-1-107-41921-6 Paperback

EDITORS' PREFACE

IN view of the increasing importance of the study of public hygiene and the recognition by doctors, teachers, administrators and members of Public Health and Hygiene Committees alike that the *salus populi* must rest, in part at least, upon a scientific basis, the Syndics of the Cambridge University Press have decided to publish a series of volumes dealing with the various subjects connected with Public Health.

The books included in the Series present in a useful and handy form the knowledge now available in many branches of the subject. They are written by experts, and the authors are occupied, or have been occupied, either in investigations connected with the various themes or in their application and administration. They include the latest scientific and practical information offered in a manner which is not too technical. The bibliographies contain references to the literature of each subject which will ensure their utility to the specialist.

It has been the desire of the editors to arrange that the books should appeal to various classes of readers : and it is hoped that they will be useful to the medical profession at home and abroad, to bacteriologists and laboratory students, to municipal engineers and architects, to medical officers of health and sanitary inspectors and to teachers and administrators.

Many of the volumes will contain material which will be suggestive and instructive to members of Public Health and Hygiene Committees ; and it is intended that they shall seek to influence the large body of educated and intelligent public opinion interested in the problems of public health.

AUTHOR'S PREFACE

OF the many subjects which at present claim attention none is more interesting or calls more insistently for our consideration than the influence of occupation upon health. The prosperity of a nation is intimately bound up with the health of the people who compose it. Recent years have witnessed improvements in the conditions under which labour is carried on in this and other countries. Factory legislation has accomplished much, much yet remains to be done. While our hearts are no longer saddened by tales of children of tender years lifted from their bed and carried in the early morning into a coal mine to spend several hours a day in darkness minding a trap door, there are still children who to-day in brickfield and factory are forced to carry weights far beyond their strength and who, as a consequence, suffer in health and remain stunted in growth.

This book has been written not for members of the medical profession alone, but for all who are interested in those movements which make for better health of the large army of workers. It ought to appeal to students of social problems and of subjects connected with public health, also to workers in the cause of industrial legislation. The space allotted is only sufficient to allow of merely the fringe of some of the subjects being reached, but even the little which has been attempted may be enough to stimulate some of the readers to take up and assist in solving problems which are of vital importance to the working classes.

As the book was partly on the way before the war began I have not thought it desirable to alter the text nor to change the references. When the war is over new labour difficulties will arise, and new social aspirations will have to be considered and met. Work, for example, will have to be found for many of the soldiers who are maimed or otherwise, and to women some consideration will have to be shown for the promptitude with which they stepped into the breach and helped their country in her hour of trial and at a time when male labour was becoming unprocurable.

THOMAS OLIVER.

Newcastle-upon-Tyne
December, 1915.

CONTENTS

ILLUSTRATIONS

INTRODUCTORY

Occupation and health: how to secure the one and maintain the other are questions which concern most of us. Before proceeding to discuss the influence of harmful trades upon man and his surroundings it might be well to pass in rapid review the origin and rise of commerce and manufacture and the interposition of the State in regard to persons employed in manufacture and industry.

There was nothing in the industrial life of the old nations akin to the factory system of to-day. Next to hunting and fishing, man's earliest occupation so long as he followed a nomadic life, must have been that of herding and rearing cattle, while to woman fell the task of looking after the family and the immediate wants of the home. Tilling of the soil was man's first settled occupation. Thus is it that agriculture is the oldest industry. Although Great Britain has long ceased to be agricultural, yet even in this country agriculture is a more important industry than most people imagine. The total number of occupied persons in the United Kingdom in 1901 was 15,388,501 (viz. 12,134,259 males and 3,254,242 females). Of this number the largest percentage 12·66 were employed in agriculture, 11·39 in commerce, 8·2 in conveyance, 7·89 in metals and machinery, 6·92 in textile fabrics, 6·77 in building and construction, and 5 per cent. in mines and quarries—that is to say, the number of persons employed in agriculture was, in 1901, nearly equal to the combined number of persons employed in the iron and metal industries and in the mines and quarries.

If there is one important difference in the industries of older nations compared with those of modern times, it is that the bulk of their work was done by slaves. It is stated that in the best days of Greece there were in Athens alone 100,000 slaves, and when Rome was reaching the height of her power, slaves formed a large proportion of the population. At this period new forces were coming to birth within the Empire. Trade and commerce had arisen, and while these were regarded with disfavour by the landed proprietors, the trading classes were gradually rising to power through the wealth they were accumulating. As Rome grew so did capitalism rise in influence. With the rise of capitalism agriculture lessened and the smaller peasantry disappeared. Slave labour supplanted that of free men on the land. Although ceasing to be a producer, Rome yet became the market of the world, and, like London to-day, the centre of Exchange. Flourishing on business she had not created, finance and banking became the features of Roman life and activity. With the rise of capitalism a new class was created, a class conscious of its power through the wealth it held, and as this class felt itself capable of directing the affairs of Empire, from it were taken its able men to fill the offices of State. In this epitome of Rome we see how trade, commerce and capitalism preceded manufacture.

Something akin to this has taken place in Great Britain. Land is still regarded as the main source of national wealth. With the rise of capitalism the commercial classes have competed with the aristocracy for power, while from their ranks the nobility has been recruited. For the last century the capitalist and commercial classes have made the largest numbers of our laws but within recent years a new power, political and social, has arisen which would hardly have been possible had it not been for the modern factory system.

With the invention of machinery and the utilization of water power, Great Britain broke loose from old methods and started on a career of her own which the introduction of steam and the wealth of her coal fields enabled her to embark upon. People also migrated into the towns where labour was cheap and abundant.

As a consequence of this industrial evolution handicrafts disappeared. The cottage method of production in which members of one family joined together for a common end was replaced by a combined system under which there was a directing head as in modern factory management. In isolated handicrafts; the result of a man's labour was his own, but in the factory system this can never be, for a workman is a unit among hundreds and is in consequence of the division of labour only a part contributor to the finished product. In the industrial handicraft of bygone years a workman impressed his personality upon the product, but in modern factory work this is impossible, for not only is production partitioned, but the work is so organized that whether the individual goes to the factory or not, the machinery runs all the same and manufacture proceeds independently of him. It would be erroneous to say that machinery has quite supplanted the brain and hands, and destroyed entirely the individuality of the worker, for some men and women can get out of machinery more than others, but although deft hands and subtle brains are still required of factory operatives, it cannot be denied that the monotony of modern factory life has dwarfed individuality, developed a kind of fatigue unknown to the working classes of two centuries ago and a longing for excitement and re-creation as a counterpoise to the depressing effects of work.

The fatigue experienced by the modern factory hand is not that which follows hard muscular work in the open air; its causation is different: into it there enter greater mental strain, the influence of work carried on in over-heated, moist and imperfectly ventilated rooms, also the noise of machinery. At first it was believed that machinery would lighten human labour. To such an extent in the early years of last century did this appear to be the case, since it seemed as if machinery could be so easily tended, that it drew into the factory not only a large amount of unskilled labour but also that of women and children as well. The first effect of machinery is to displace labour: fewer hands are required, but as man's wants keep increasing, and machine made goods cost less and do not wear so well, production is in the end stimulated so that in the end a larger number of persons find employment. With the introduction of machinery has come unregulated competition to which, and to over-production, many of our modern industrial troubles are attributed.

In the early part of the 19th century England awoke to a realisation of the injustice and the injury which were being done to child life by over-work in the mills, the unwholesome conditions under which work was carried on, the equally wretched conditions under which the apprenticed children were housed and fed, to say nothing of the uncalled for cruelty of their masters. The bringing of a man named Jouvaux to justice in 1801 for ill-treating and over-working his 16 apprentices, of providing these unhappy children with only two beds, of keeping them when at work in such attitudes that the children ran the risk of becoming deformed and disabled for life, wrung from the Judge on the bench remarks which find an echo in our heart to-day, that if trade cannot be carried on without children's lives being sacrificed to Moloch, men and women being slowly done to death or ruined in life and body, then such trade must be abolished.

The intentions of those who passed the Elizabethan Poor Law of 1601 may have been good, since the law directed that destitute children and orphans should be apprenticed to some trade. In establishing homes of industry wherein children should be instructed in spinning and weaving, charity found an outlet for her energy, but the system agreed upon was open to abuse. Under well conditioned circumstances life could have been made not only bearable, but pleasurable for the children, but the long hours 6 to 6 in summer and 7 to 5 in winter, with compulsory attendance at evening classes when the day's work was done, robbed childhood of all that belonged to it and was hardly likely to be followed by a sturdy manhood and strong womanhood. The treatment of pauper children, the disregard of child life and of its claims to protection, the evils of compulsory apprenticeship, overcrowding and the want of education, form the dark side of the "Industrial Revolution." When events became more widely known and it was felt that masters and overseers had failed in their duty towards child labour and treatment of the young, the public conscience was awakened and a new mental attitude was assumed towards industrial questions which could only be calmed by legislation. It was in 1802 that the first Act which regulated labour in factories was passed. This, known as the "Factory Health and Morals Act" of 1802, and spoken of as the elder Sir Robert Peel's Act, was rather an extension of the old Poor Law than an attempt to assume control over industry.

This Act limited the power of work for apprentices to 12 hours per day: night work was to be gradually dropped: the children were to receive a certain amount of education and were to be given one suit of clothes yearly: better sleeping accommodation was to be provided: attendance at church once a month was compulsory: a form of inspection by the local authority was instituted and factories were to be registered. Subsequently as factory owners began to find inspection irksome, free children's labour was introduced and it gradually replaced that of the apprentices who had been drawn from the workhouses and industrial homes.

What those dark days of apprenticeship meant imagination alone can supply. The cry of the children however had been heard, but it was not till 1819 that an Act was passed which limited the age to 9, at which work should begin in the factories. No young person under the age of 16 was to be employed more than 12 hours a day, exclusive of meal time. The principal point in the Act was the prohibition of child labour under 9. It still left the inspection of the factories and of the children in the hands of local Justices although experience of the previous Act had shown how impracticable the whole system was. The Act of 1819 was followed by a short amending Act which allowed time lost by such an accident as water failure to be made up by working overtime or in the night, also, by doing away with a fixed time for dinner so that this meal became a moveable feast to be partaken of at any time between 11 a.m. and 4 p.m. instead of 11 and 2. As Miss Hutchins says in her admirable *History of Factory Legislation*, from which I have freely quoted, this was a retrograde step. The Act of 1825 reduced the working day by 1½ hours: it fixed the dinner hour between 11 and 2, and it limited Saturday labour to 9 hours. To enable some factories to close earlier on Saturday work had to be begun at 5 o'clock in the morning.

In 1831 when Michael Sadler introduced into Parliament his Ten Hours' Bill, factory life was anything but satisfactory. The hours were long, the atmosphere of the rooms was overheated, children were still subjected to indignity and cruelty, no opportunity was given for education nor time for play and recreation. Many of the young workers under 18 years of age were not employed directly by the owners of the factory but by the operatives themselves. There was a tendency therefore for a father to employ his own children and to exploit them for profit. The Factory Act of 1833 was in advance of its predecessors, for it prohibited in cotton mills and other factories night work to all persons under 18 years of age, while child labour under 9 was abolished. No child under 11 years of age could be employed for more than 9 hours a day. During meal hours, children were not allowed to remain in the room with the machinery. Four factory inspectors were appointed with power to enter factories at any time, to examine the children and to make any enquiry they thought necessary.

From 1841–1847 women's labour was the subject of discussion. The increasing employment of women in factories had become a source of uneasiness to many of the social reformers who were of the opinion that in the home lay the true vocation of woman. Those men therefore were disposed to limit the number of female operatives and to prohibit married women working in the mills so long as their husbands were alive and earning an income.

A 10 hours' day had been secured for the working classes by the Act of 1847. From that date onward to 1860 little was effected in the way of factory legislation. Although it was for the textile trades that most of the legislation had been passed, yet by degrees other industries were brought within the law. Children of tender years were being employed in potteries—their hours were long and the work was irregular. In consequence of the nature of the employment and the high temperature to which the workers were exposed, 120° to 140° F., it was apparent that there was occurring among the workers a physical degeneracy, each succeeding generation it was said had become more dwarfed and less robust than its predecessor.

The Act of 1864 gave better definition of a factory and required that factories were to be kept clean and that gases detrimental to health were to be removed. By the Workshops' Regulation Act of 1867 the Local Authorities were made responsible for the administration of the law in workshops, but this Act was a failure. Under the Act neither a Medical Officer of Health nor an Inspector under the Local Authority could enter a workshop without an order from a Justice empowering him to do so within 48 hours after the date of issue of the order. There were no sanitary provisions contained in the Act; these followed in the Sanitary Act of 1896.

Space will not permit of the various items of Factory Legislation being dealt with in detail. The aims and objects of recent factory legislation are closely associated with the spirit and practice of the Employers' Liability Act and the Workmen's Compensation Act, so that employers and employed are brought frequently into opposition. There has been a growing conviction that each industry should bear the burden of the misfortunes it creates. It is hardly fair that a fatal accident occurring in the course of employment, and which deprives a family of its bread winner, should be allowed to bring absolute poverty into a home and deprive wife and children of the means of subsistence. It has only been by degrees that certain diseases caused through occupation, and which are consequences of it, have come to be regarded in the same light as accidents and entitling to compensation. Much of the recent factory and social legislation has been anticipated by the work done by Departmental Committees and Commissions.

Factory legislation will always be objected to by many persons on the grounds that it is an interference with the liberty of the subject, but as the social organization has become more complete, the units composing it have become more and more interdependent. Man does not live to himself alone. In all dangerous occupations, workpeople cannot be left entirely to their own devices, nor can they be allowed to take chances. It was thus that at its inception factory legislation dealt with child labour since children are unable to take care of themselves: subsequently it concerned itself with women's work owing to the absence of labour organization and the fact that it was to women as possible mothers that reformers looked for the perpetuation of a race worthy of the country in which its units are born. Factory employment has been both a gain and a loss to the nation. The gains are generally admitted to outweigh the losses. One of the drawbacks to it is the withdrawal into its service of a large army of young women whose life might be spent at home with greater benefit to the race and with more influence for good upon the family. Factory legislation is, in its objects, humane. It recognizes that life and limb must be protected and that in the case of death or accident employment carries with it financial responsibilities over and above the wages given for services rendered.

BIBLIOGRAPHY

Hutchins, Miss B. L. *History of Factory Legislation.*
Taylor, Whateley Cooke. *Modern Factory System.* Kegan Paul, 1891.

CHAPTER I

THE AIR WE BREATHE IN TOWN AND COUNTRY. AIR IN THE NEIGHBOURHOOD OF FACTORIES. INFLUENCE OF SMOKE. DUST, TRAFFIC AND MICRO-ORGANISMS

Statistics show that the healthiest life man can lead is that spent in the open air. The longevity of the agricultural classes is some compensation for their exclusion from the excitement incidental to living in towns. Rural depopulation and the rise of large towns are the inevitable consequences of the changes which have taken place in our industrial methods. Factories have changed environment, some of the quiet country towns of a century ago are to-day hives of industry. Coal mines and iron works have altered localities. Travelling by rail one passes from pastoral and wooded scenery into districts where the stunted trees and scanty vegetation give evidence of the struggle nature has had with the unhealthy influences created by the industrial activity of man. Some modern trade developments poison the atmosphere, while the refuse of dye works and the washing of mineral ores pollute the rivers and kill the fish. In the vicinity of chemical works vegetation is well nigh impossible. Exposed to chemical emanations the tops of trees decay. In the immediate neighbourhood of coke ovens trees become blighted and cease to put on leaf. Animals grazing near lead smelting works have died from plumbism, and birds which have eaten berries grown in the neighbourhood of lead smelting works have shared a similar fate. Last year (1914) while visiting a large zinc and lead smelting works on the continent, the manager informed me that the ducks which used to swim in the canal adjoining the works had become paralysed in their legs and could no longer paddle. A few months after my visit to the Trabonelli sulphur mine in Sicily, an explosion occurred in the mine—several lives were lost. For several months afterwards the gases which escaped from the mine were of such a poisonous nature that birds flying over the plant fell down dead.

The death of two horses on a farm near Swansea in December 1912, also of another since, and which formed the subject of a special enquiry, was found to have been the result of the animals having grazed where fumes from spelter works had become deposited. In the stomach of the animals the county analyst found 0·16 grain of lead, 0·009 grain of arsenic and 1·0 grain of zinc. Cattle grazing in the immediate neigh-bourhood of the Broken Hill mines in Australia died from lead poisoning, fowls could not be reared, and in one instance a child died from plumbism due to having sucked flowers upon some of which was found lead. Cases such as these show the risks which man and animals are exposed to in eating uncooked and unwashed vegetables grown in the neighbour-hood of spelter and lead smelting works, also of the necessity of capturing by some means or other the fumes so that they shall not escape into the open air and poison man and beast. It is just possible that some of the ill-health of persons living in the immediate neighbourhood of large smelting works may be due to minute metallic particles being inhaled or swallowed with the food. It is a mistake to have dwelling houses too near slag and furnace refuse heaps for on several occasions poisonous gases, chiefly carbon monoxide, have penetrated the soil and reaching the cottages have caused death of some of the inmates.

Excess of coal smoke is a cause of a high death rate from acute diseases of the respiratory organs. To this subject Dr Louis Ascher of Königsberg has given attention. He found that while the mortality from tuberculosis among coal miners was low both in Prussia and England, he was surprised to find that the mortality from acute lung diseases, other than those of a tuberculous nature, was high. In manufacturing countries the highest mortality from acute lung disease is found in those districts where coal smoke is most abundant. Smoke not only tends to produce pulmonary disease but it hastens the course of tuberculosis. Ascher's experiments on this point are of interest. He caused (1) rabbits to inhale coal smoke and then infected them by getting the animals to breathe such an organism as *aspergillus fumigatus*: (2) other rabbits were infected by *aspergillus fumigatus* without breathing coal smoke: (3) rabbits were infected with tubercle and inhaled coal smoke, while (4) others were similarly infected but not exposed to coal smoke. The infected animals which inhaled coal smoke died on an average 53 days after the commencement of the experiment, whereas the infected animals which did not inhale smoke lived for 90 days. It is not for the moment maintained that in industrial districts coal smoke is the only adverse factor in causing a high death rate from acute respiratory disease. There are such additional circumstances as climate, nature of occupation, home life and surroundings, infection, e.g. influenza, also alcohol which cannot be ignored. That fine particles of mineral and other forms of dust predispose to pneumonia, allusion need only be made to the high death rate from pneumonia among the native races working on the Rand, the slag workers in Germany and the labourers in the iron works of Middlesbrough.

The uncontrolled escape of smoke from factories is an economic waste. This, as well as the escape of chemical vapours and emanation of disagreeable gases, should be prevented as far as possible.

Man can become accustomed to almost everything including noise. People living in houses close to large works cease to be influenced by noise, but in times of illness especially of a nervous nature they recover more quickly if removed to a quieter home. On account of noise, day and night, also the danger of fire, dwelling-houses should not abut upon factories nor should they be situated near places where large quantities of petrol and benzol are stored, dry cleaning of goods carried on, nor where celluloid is manufactured, as during the combustion of celluloid prussic acid is evolved and is dangerous.

The proximity of rag and bone stores to dwelling-houses is not in keeping with the laws of health. Tanneries, slaughter houses, places where rabbit skins are cleaned, also where grease is boiled are undesirable in overcrowded districts. Similar remarks apply to guano, phospho-guano and nitrogenous superphosphate stores. From all of these unpleasant odours are given off which cannot but contribute to deranging digestion and destroying taste for food.

Not only may gas, fume and dust pollute the atmosphere in the neighbourhood of a factory, but micro-organisms may be present in the air as well. Anthrax or wool sorters' disease is due to a specific microbe. Cattle which had grazed on pasture land adjoining a wool factory in Yorkshire died from anthrax due to dust given off during the opening of bales of infected wool and wafted from the factory into the outside air by the currents created by the running of fans.

The air of large towns contains numerous micro-organisms. Upon most of them the ultra-violet rays of the sun have a distinctly bactericidal influence, hence micro-organisms are usually more numerous in the shade than in the sunlight. During rainy weather the number of micro-organisms in the air diminishes. They are washed down into the soil. In dried expectoration taken from a pavement in Birmingham Dr John Robertson found tubercle bacilli. Dry sweeping of streets raises clouds of dust along with micro-organisms into the air. To this circumstance is attributed by Mr Frederick L. Hoffman of the Prudential Assurance Society of America the great amount of sickness and the high death rate from pulmonary phthisis which until lately prevailed among the street sweepers of New York. Street dust contains in addition to tubercle bacilli other pathogenic organisms such as the *bacillus coli*, *bacillus aerogenes capsulatus* and many varieties of cocci. To the pollen of certain plants, floating in the air as fine dust, is due the hay fever to which certain persons are especially susceptible. Apart from that evolved from chimneys, dust in the streets may have been wind-borne from a considerable distance. Street dust is added to during the demolition of old houses: it is raised into the atmosphere by passing traffic and particularly so owing to the increase of motor car and steam lorry traffic. Increased amounts of dust raised into the air are accompanied by a corresponding rise in the number of micro-organisms. Air taken from a street in front of the Madeline in Paris in the summer of 1911 when examined by MM. Sartory and Langlais contained at

8 a.m.	...	545 bacteria per cm.	
10 a.m.	...	2,300	,,	,,
midday	...	9,600	,,	,,
2 p.m.	...	14,200	,,	,,
5 p.m.	...	20,800	,,	,,

Air taken in the Place de la Concorde contained at

7 a.m.	...	640 bacteria per cm.	
10 a.m.	...	780	,,	,,
11 a.m.	...	1,800	,,	,,
midday	...	23,000	,,	,,
2 p.m.	...	72,000	,,	,,
4 p.m.	...	75,000	,,	,,
6 p.m.	...	80,000	,,	,,
7 p.m.	...	88,000	,,	,,

From the above it will be seen that in throwing up dust into the air, traffic at the same time increases the number of bacteria. Street dust and bacteria are not lifted high into the atmosphere. At the top of the Pantheon only 28 bacteria per cm. of air were found, and at the top of the tower of Notre Dame 40 per cm. At the top of the Clock Tower of the Houses of Parliament in London, Graham Smith found only one-third of the number of bacteria which he found at the ground level. Although it is estimated that a person living in London inhales 300,000 microbes daily, fortunately they belong to the harmless varieties and come from the soil. The micro-organisms which are harmful come from man and from the lower animals and are thrown off in the excreta.

As illustrating the pollution of the atmosphere which takes place during the demolition of houses, air taken from the Avenue de l'Opera contained 500 to 10,000 bacteria per cm. but in air taken close to a house which was being pulled down the number of bacteria in the same volume of air varied from 112,000 to 240,000. All this shows the necessity of workmen playing the hose so as to lay dust with water during the demolition of houses. The dust given off is not only harmful to the men employed but as it penetrates into adjoining houses and shops it is a nuisance for it destroys goods.

Country villages hitherto healthy to live in on account of their inaccessibility and comparative freedom from dust are being invaded by the motor car while agricultural land which borders upon the highways is having its yield curtailed by dust from the roads. The dust raised by passing automobiles is harmful to pedestrians with delicate lungs on account of its contained siliceous particles: it is equally a source of annoyance and discomfort to cottagers by the wayside who are obliged to keep their windows and front door closed. On a road leading from Ville d'Avray while the number of bacteria per cm. varied on week days from 190 to 215, on Sundays when motor cars were passing, almost without cessation, Sartory and Langlais found that the numbers rose to 538,000 and even to 910,000. The bacteria on the road to St Cloud, a popular drive from Paris, numbered on week days 320 to 890 per cm. of air, but on Sundays they were present to the extent of 328,000 to 670,000 per cm. of air. These observations are of further interest since some were made of air taken over parts of the road which had been tarred, others on parts which had not been so dealt with. Air taken at 10–11 a.m. on a week day from a tarred part of the road in the Avenue St Cloud gave 19,000 bacteria per cm. and air from a non-tarred portion contained 610,000 micro-organisms: at 4–5 p.m., air removed from a tarred part of the road gave 72,000 and that from a non-tarred portion 1,800,000. On Sundays when there is much motor traffic, air taken from a tarred portion of the road gave between 10–11 a.m. 2,200,000 per cm., that from a non-tarred portion 7,220,000, while between 4–5 p.m. the numbers were 4,250,000 and 12,000,000 respectively. The Avenue St Cloud was chosen by MM. Sartory and Langlais on account of the great motor traffic upon it.

Tarring of the roads, contrary to the opinions expressed by many persons and the dry throats which it is said to cause, has therefore a beneficial influence not only as regards the amount of dust raised but upon the health of the people as well. In some factories tarring of the main roads inside the works has been followed by a reduction in the amount of respiratory disease especially among young workers. The average sick rate, 30 per cent., fell to 12 per cent. after tarring was introduced. While tarring of roads has in some instances been beneficial in others it has been harmful. It has destroyed vegetation and the dust blown into rivers has spoiled them for angling purposes.

A simple method of determining the amount of dust in air is to allow the dust to settle upon a Petri dish. Particles of dust can thereafter be examined under the microscope or gathered upon a watch glass and weighed. To weigh air, a quantity measured in a gas meter must be passed through cotton or some other filtering material and the filter weighed afterwards. The quantity of air used should be large so that the amount of dust may be appreciable. The filtering material is weighed both before the air has passed through it and afterwards. As increase in weight of the filter might be due to absorption of water this must be guarded against by placing the filtering material in a desiccator before and after filtration and weighing in each instance.

For determining bacteria in the air *The Bacteriological examination of food and water* by Dr W. G. Savage (Cambridge Public Health Series) should be consulted.

BIBLIOGRAPHY

Robertson, John, M.D. *Health Reports, City of Birmingham.*
Louis Ascher, Dr. *Journal of the Royal Sanitary Institute*, vol. XXVIII, No. 2, 1907.
Hoffman, Frederick L. *Mortality from Consumption and Dusty Trades.*
A. Sartory and M. Langlais. *Poussières et Microbes de l'Air.* A. Binat, Editeur. Paris, 1912.

CHAPTER II

THE AIR OF FACTORIES, WORKSHOPS AND WORKROOMS. DUSTY WORKSHOPS. TUBERCULOSIS AND LUNG DISEASES. VENTILATION AND STERILIZATION OF THE AIR. INFLUENCE OF TOBACCO SMOKE IN CLEARING THE AIR

Important as is the air of the home from a health point of view, that of the factory and workroom is equally so since working men and women are obliged to spend several hours a day therein under conditions which frequently impose a burden upon the respiratory organs and the skin. If not renewed sufficiently the air of a factory and workshop is rendered impure by the products given off by the lungs and skin of the work-people themselves, by the products of the incomplete combustion of artificial illuminants, by gases evolved and dust given off during the manufacture of certain products or from materials used in processes of manufacture. In order that air may be health-promoting it must be kept circulating. It is when air is stagnant, contains an excess of carbon dioxide and of proteid material, that it ceases to be vitalizing. Work-people inhaling day after day impure air become anaemic and prone to illness. We attach less importance to slight excesses of carbon dioxide in the air of workrooms than did physiologists half a century ago. In exhaled air there are other things than carbon dioxide, water and traces of proteid: from the skin and intestinal canal there escape gases all of which unitedly give rise to the peculiar odour characteristic of a close room.

The amount of carbon dioxide present is regarded as a measure of the vitiation of the air. Proust thought the air of a room close if it contained 7 parts of carbon dioxide per 10,000. The Commission which sat in England in 1896 to consider the operations of the Cotton Cloth Act of 1889 admitted that while it might be thought the amount was too high from a medical point of view, yet recommended that the air of workrooms should not contain more than 9 volumes of carbon dioxide per 10,000. There should be constant renewal of the air so that each person should be able to command 32 cubic metres of air per hour. The French Commission of Industrial Hygiene, which sat in 1906, expressed the opinion that conditions were not satisfactory in any place where work was carried on whenever the amount of carbon dioxide in the atmosphere exceeded 10 volumes per 10,000, but this was not to apply to places where carbon dioxide is given off into the air during industrial operations and the examination made when the workrooms are lighted artificially unless by electricity. The purity of air depends less upon the spatial cubic capacity than upon the quantity of air introduced and its renewal.

The dusty atmosphere of a workroom is equally obnoxious. The part played by dust in causing ill-health has long been recognized. Dust is injurious in several ways. It may be a direct poison as in the case of white lead and arsenic: it may be injurious to the lungs on account of the hard and spiky character of the particles it carries or it may be risky to life on account of its explosive character. Dust generated in factories is organic, like flour and cotton, or it is inorganic like lead, steel and emery. Frequently there are germs adherent to the particles of dust and thereby another danger is superadded.

To the group of diseases caused by dust a French physician, Layet, gave the name of *nosoconioses*. According to the tissues or organs affected *nosoconioses* are subdivided into *pneumoconioses* or dust affection of the lungs, *enteroconioses* when the gastro-intestinal tract is implicated, *rhinoconioses* the nose and throat, *dermatoconioses* the skin, and *ophthalmoconioses* the eye. Apart from maladies of an infectious nature also those due to subacute poisoning, such as plumbism, the diseases of the lungs caused by dust are the most important. An association which must not be lost sight of is that of Tuberculosis and dusty occupations, also to what extent the one predisposes to the other. *Pneumoconiosis* or occupational phthisis can be caused by breathing dust alone but as the illness proceeds, infection may become superadded, so that a pulmonary lesion which at its inception was non-tuberculous may subsequently become tuberculous. The change in the character of the disease may be due to the inhalation of tubercle bacilli from the dried expectoration of a consumptive fellow workman.

It is not insisted upon that a tuberculous workman should not be allowed to take his place as hitherto in factory or workshop, but men or women who are the subjects of pulmonary tuberculosis would, for their own sakes, be better out of the dusty atmosphere of a workroom. The spread of tuberculosis in a workroom can be prevented by free ventilation, abundance of daylight and of air space, and by requiring that all workmen who are the subjects of chronic cough shall expectorate into spittoons distributed throughout the factory and which not only contain disinfectants but are emptied and disinfected daily. No dry sweeping of the floors should be attempted during the hours of work or shortly before work commences. The floors sprinkled with a disinfecting fluid should be swept at the close of the day when the workpeople have left the workrooms. By sweeping the floor in the evening any dust which has been raised into the air will have settled down again by the morning.

Sartory and Langlais have estimated the possible amount of mineral and vegetable dust a workman may receive into his system during 10 hours of work in the following occupations:

> 0·10 grm of dust in a saw mill.
> 0·12 ,,   ,,   in an iron foundry.
> 1·08 grms   ,,   during the grinding of phosphates.
> 1·12 ,,   ,,   in a cement works.

Arens supplies the following data as regards dust per cm. of air removed from workrooms:

> 15 to 17 mgrms in saw mills during work.
> 22 to 28 ,,   in grinding mills with three crushing machines in operation.
> 130 mgrms in cement works during absence of workmen.
> 224 ,,   in cement works when two grinding mills are in operation.

Among dusty trades may be mentioned the cleaning of bales of raw cotton, hemp and jute, emptying of the stacks in white lead factories, certain processes of china and earthenware manufacture, cutlery and file making. In my book, *Diseases of Occupation*, I draw attention to the fact that in the manufacture of earthenware the air, in which brushers-off, porcelain makers, and finishers carry on their work, frequently contains 640 million particles of dust per cubic metre of air, while several of the finishers, those persons whose work consists in removing the excess of the dried glaze on the ware may be found breathing an atmosphere containing 680 million particles of dust per cm. of air. All grinding trades are more or less dusty. In one cubic metre of air Hesse found:

> In a felt hat factory ... ...   175 mgrms of dust.
> In an old flour mill ... ...   48 ,,   ,,
> In a new flour mill ... ...   4 ,,   ,,
> In an iron works ... ...   72–100 mgrms of dust.
> In a coal mine ... ...   14 mgrms of dust.

These tables give details as to amounts of dust which might be inhaled but it is not contended for one moment that all the dust reaches the lungs for there are many obstacles, physical and physiological, to prevent it reaching the pulmonary alveoli. In addition to dust, micro-organisms, and such moulds as aspergilli and mucors, may also be inhaled. During the opening out of bales of horse hair in horse hair factories considerable quantities of dust escape into the air. In a cubic metre of air taken from a room where bales of horse hair were being opened 4 to 9 million bacteria were found. In addition to the various types of bacilli such organisms as *staphylococcus pyogenes aureus, penicilium glaucum, mucor mucedo* and *flavus* were found. On one occasion anthrax bacilli with *staphylococci* and *streptococci* were found. A culture of the anthrax bacilli was made and injected into a rabbit and a guinea pig with the result that both animals died, and from the blood removed from the heart a culture of *bacillus anthracis* was obtained. In air taken from other factories wherein wool-fleeces were being opened 182,200 micro-organisms per cm. were obtained. Among these were included *staphylococci, streptococci* and the *pneumobacillus* of Friedländer. It is a fortunate circumstance that so many of the microbes in the air are non-pathogenic and non-virulent.

During the sorting of feathers and the unpacking of the down of geese the air becomes dusty and micro-organisms are frequently present in great numbers. Before bales of hair, wool, feather or down are opened they ought to be disinfected by being exposed to dry heat or steam, otherwise illness among the workers may supervene. Even where no such serious disease as anthrax follows the mere complaint of headache, acute abdominal pain and gastric derangement with vomiting or retching are enough to show that the individual has inhaled something out of the usual. Tame pigeons and domesticated birds are liable to the malady known as "tuberculosis aspergillaris," and as the mould, *aspergillus fumigatus*, is the cause of the disease and is frequently present in the dust given off during the sorting and cleaning of feathers, disinfection of the bales of feathers before opening them in a factory is a wise and safe procedure.

How to purify the air of factories is no easy task. Improve the ventilation by introducing and causing more air to circulate at once suggests itself. The objection to natural ventilation by the open window is that it never can be depended upon. It is irregular: it often creates a good deal of discomfort and the workpeople frequently complain of the cold and draughts. Briefly expressed, ventilation by the open window is either insufficient or it is in excess. The running of a fan which only creates currents without an escape for the air is of no use. It only raises dust into the air but does not remove it. The sprinkling of floors with water and disinfectants after the day's work is done is useful. One method of disinfecting air is to pass it through an electrical sterilisator. The sterilisator rapidly destroys germ life. In the case of a workroom, of 100 cubic metres capacity, and in the air of which there were at first 40,000 to 50,000 bacteria per cm. after 1 hour's treatment of the air by the sterilisator the number of micro-organisms fell to 10,000 per cm.: in 2 hours to 1000 and after 3 hours the air was found to have been rendered completely sterile, the interesting point being that all this was accomplished without the temperature being raised more than 3° C.

In carrying out a series of experiments with fine bronze powder in a laboratory through which a strong beam of light made a brilliantly illuminated pathway, it seemed to other observers in the room as well as myself that tobacco smoke from a pipe or cigarette when brought into contact with the dust floating in the air cleared the atmosphere much more quickly than if the dust was allowed to settle alone. The circumstance is interesting not only because in tobacco smoke we have a possible means of clearing the dusty atmosphere of a room, but also on account of the fact that as in the nose of persons who use snuff and in the mouth of smokers fewer bacteria are found than in the nose and mouth of persons who neither snuff nor smoke, tobacco smoke after all may possess bactericidal properties. Microbes cannot live in water in which tobacco has been steeped. In the interior of cigars no bacteria are found. According to Dr Wenck, Professor of the Imperial Institute, Berlin, cholera microbes die in from one half to two hours after exposure to tobacco smoke. During an epidemic of cholera in Hamburg, Wenck did not find a single cigar maker attacked by the disease.

Attention to the nasal passages is highly necessary in persons who are working in dusty processes especially where the dust is of an organic nature.

Of pathogenic microbes the one which is the most active cause of suppuration is *staphylococcus pyogenes aureus*. It is prevalent in industrial dust of organic origin. The microbe tends to lurk in the nostrils of those who inhale the dust or it invades the lachrymal duct and becomes a cause of conjunctivitis.

In dusty trades the micro-organism which is so provocative of harm is the tubercle bacillus. Tatham tells us that there are 22 industries in each of which the mortality from tuberculous phthisis and respiratory diseases together is more than double that of agriculturists. Taking the mortality ratio of agriculturists as 100, potters give a ratio of 453, cutlers 407, file makers 373, glass makers 335, iron and steel workers 292, lead workers 247, and workers in cotton mills 244. If we turn to German statistics we find in a similar manner that the incidence of pulmonary tuberculosis varies with the nature of the occupation. Sommerfeld gives the following as the proportion of persons per thousand in the various dusty occupations who die of pulmonary tuberculosis.

Occupation unattended by dust production	...	2·39
,, with dust production	... ...	5·42
,, ,, iron dust	... ...	5·55
,, ,, lead dust	... ...	7·79
,, ,, tobacco dust	... ...	8·47
,, ,, porcelain dust	... ...	14·0
,, ,, stone dust	... ...	34·9

Frederick L. Hoffman reproduces some interesting figures bearing upon this question. In men whose occupation exposes them to metallic dust the proportion of deaths from consumption at ages 15–24 is 46·5 per cent., at ages 25–34 it is 57·2 per cent., at ages 35–44 it is 42·4 per cent., and at ages 45–54 it is 23·4 per cent. As regards men exposed in their occupation to mineral dust the facts are not quite so serious. The mortality from consumption at the ages of 15–24 is 31·7 per cent., at 25–34, 47·6 per cent., at 35–44, 36·3 per cent., and at the ages of 45–54 it is 27·9 per cent. When we turn our attention to steel grinders we are struck by the high mortality from pulmonary consumption. Between the ages of 25 and 34 it is 70·8 per cent. as against 31·3 per cent. for men in all occupations. Such is the toll exacted of men who work in occupations the air of which contains dust.

BIBLIOGRAPHY

A. Sartory and M. Langlais. *Poussières et Microbes de l'Air.* Binat, Paris, 1912.

Oliver, Thomas. *Diseases of Occupation.* Methuen and Co., London.

Oliver, Thomas. *Maladies caused by the Air we breathe.* Baillière. Tindall and Cox.

Tatham, John. *Dangerous Trades.* Edited by Thomas Oliver. John Murray, London.

Hoffman, Frederick L. "Influence of Trades on Disease." *Proc. Ninth Annual Congress of Sanitary Officers of the State of New York,* 1909.

CHAPTER III

WORK, WAGES, EFFICIENCY AND FATIGUE. MACHINERY AND SPEEDING UP. SWEATED INDUSTRIES. ARTIFICIAL FLOWER MAKING. FEATHER CLEANING

While labour saving machinery is supposed to lighten toil, it frequently imposes a fresh burden upon the physical powers and the endurance of workers. Sixty years ago when hand loom weaving was still a home industry men worked during their own time and in accordance with their inclination. Personal circumstances dictated whether throwing the shuttle was to be regarded as toil or as a leisured occupation. Factory work on the contrary equalises the conditions for all operatives since to keep pace with the running of machinery all the "hands" must work in concert. A century ago the weekly wages of a Lancashire cotton spinner were 6 shillings and 5 pence: thirty years ago they were 25 shillings, to earn which he supervised 600 spindles. At present a spinner will look after 1360 spindles and for that he receives 55 shillings a week. To earn this he is on his feet all the day long: he has to keep moving over the floor space allotted to the machinery which he tends—there is never a minute of rest except when he is mending broken threads and then it is not cessation of work but change. His nervous system is in a state of tension from the time he commences work until he finishes. Strain is known to be more exhausting than work. To strain must also be added the influence of the monotony of employment, the influence of noise and of work carried on in over-heated rooms and a humid atmosphere. As a consequence of exposure to these the men by the time they reach 60 years of age are quite unable to go on with the work and have to be given less well paid employment in the factory. In all textile factories the main object is to get out of machinery the greatest production possible, to secure which machinery has to be sped up to a degree almost impossible for human strength to cope with it for any great length of time.

In shipyards the ironplate work is so rushed that the apprentices have to run in order to keep the platers supplied with hot rivets: in their haste many of these boys during the wet weather slip on the greasy surface of the deck and are seriously injured. As the week proceeds the platers become increasingly tired and are glad to rest on Saturday afternoon and Sunday. Good wages and a quiet home in open surroundings enable workmen to throw off fatigue, but the one day of rest in the seven is that which brings the fullest recuperation.

Between night and morning there is not sufficient time always for the fatigue products of the day's work to be got rid of, and so there occurs a cumulative effect. Work done by muscle already tired is more harmful than work attempted under normal conditions. Although only a few muscles of the body may have been over-worked fatigue does not remain associated with those muscles alone. It tends to become diffused over the whole muscular system. A labourer therefore who continues to work when he is fatigued not only does less effective work but he is doing himself a physical injury. It is necessary that fatigue shall be met by rest. Recovery from over fatigue may be a slow process. It is here that the 7th day's rest comes in most helpfully. Dr Haegler by means of the accompanying chart has indicated how our vital forces are affected by work and restored by rest. In the diagram too it is seen how the night's rest is not always enough to restore sufficiently the loss for the day. The result is that the line is not quite on the same level in the morning that it was 24 hours before. The chart clearly indicates that the level of our energy is somewhat lowered day by day and is recovered by the Sunday's rest. The charts were shown by

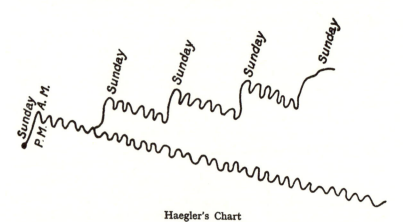

Haegler's Chart

Fatigue curves showing morning rise and afternoon depression. The upper line shows the effect of the weekly day of rest. The lower line shows the gradual depression of strength with daily work and no term of rest.

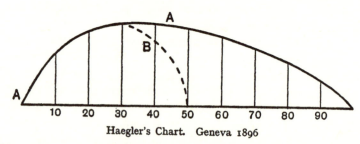

Haegler's Chart. Geneva 1896

Line A shows the normal average of life with proper time of rest. Line B shows the average life line under over-work and insufficient rest.

Haegler at the Swiss International Exposition in Geneva, 1896. The second chart shows that life is prolonged in those who take the Sunday's rest.

Equally instructive is the relation of accidents and fatigue. It is the experience of all countries that accidents increase with hours of work and that fatigue is largely responsible for them. A tired workman can no longer put forth his usual effort, nor execute movements as rapidly. Accidents take place in largest number towards the end of the forenoon, and again just before, but not quite in, the last hour of work of the afternoon. It was Germany which first introduced notification of accidents and of the period of the day at which they occurred. German statistics show that the accident rate is highest during the third and fourth hours of work. French, Belgian and British statistics, as well as those of the United States, practically speaking confirm the fact. Since the largest number of accidents is not always in the last hour before ceasing work the question has been raised, why, if fatigue is the cause of accident the number is not greatest in the last hour of work when men and women are most tired? Miss Josephine Goldmark, in her excellent treatise, attributes this partly to the variations in "quitting time" and to the fact that the first period of work is one of "limbering up" when the worker has not yet reached his normal plane of efficiency or of production. In the last hour of work production usually falls in consequence of fatigue. This circumstance of itself is not without influence in reducing the accident rate for it is in operations requiring increased speed that there tends to be produced a heightened accident rate. Owing to slackened speed in the last hour of work the accident rate falls. It is not maintained for one moment that all accidents are the result of fatigue. There are psychological as well as physiological factors which enter into their causation.

Fatigue and its place in modern Industry

The complaint of modern times is one of "feeling tired." We live in an age of fatigue, and of conditions predisposing to it. Life is lived too quickly. Occupation is exacting from workers, both mentally and physically, more than similar occupations exacted half a century ago. The causes of industrial fatigue are many: one is that too hard work may be imposed upon young persons not old enough and not sufficiently developed to bear it. As regards long hours and working overtime the trend of legislation has been to shorten the hours of labour but while this is taking place machinery is being run at greater speed in textile factories and work is being rushed in shipyards and in the iron and steel industries. The increasing number of accidents in shipyards, especially among rivetters, is largely the result of "rushing." Occasionally no explanation of an accident is found but the men themselves are of the opinion that as the result of standing too long in a strained position, and of working hard without even short intervals of rest, they become dizzy. In shipyards accidents are more frequent on Monday and Tuesday, on Friday and Saturday. Some of the accidents which occur on Monday are attributed to over-indulgence in alcohol over the week end, but some are also probably due to the men not having got quite into the swing and rhythm of the work, while as regards some of the accidents which occur on Friday and Saturday fatigue is a probable cause.

In addition to the speeding up of machinery in cotton mills the fact that the work is carried on in a warm and humid atmosphere must not be forgotten. Dr Pembrey of Guy's Hospital and Dr Edgar Collis of the Home Office have reported upon this subject. In a warm moist atmosphere not only does the pulse quicken, the skin become flushed and warm, but the temperature of the mouth rises approaching to that of the internal temperature which is also slightly raised. Weavers when at work are on their feet all day long watching for broken threads. They travel several miles daily over the floor space allotted to them, but this circumstance will hardly explain the rise of body temperature. Warm moist atmospheres reduce the differences between the internal temperature and that of the skin. While tending to establish a more uniform heat of the body generally warm moist atmospheres impose a tax upon the powers of accommodation as indicated by the low blood pressure. Muscular work raises the internal heat and up to a certain point this is an advantage to the worker. Should the air be hot and moist, more blood will be sent to the skin to be cooled, but unless perspiration takes place there will be little or no reduction of temperature. More blood sent to the skin to be cooled means more work thrown upon the heart and greater demands made upon the central nervous system to regulate the distribution of blood. When in consequence of long continued physical exertion the skin has become warmed, there occur a lowering of the muscular tone, a lessening of the exchanges of the materials of the body and a depression of the appetite. It is circumstances such as these which explain the pallor of cotton weavers, their slim build and shortness of stature, their complaint of indigestion and loss of appetite with an accompanying sense of fatigue.

Although in many respects the conditions in the manufacture of cotton and flax differ widely, in both industries the operatives are exposed to moist atmospheres often at high temperatures, the temperature in flax spinning being generally the higher. Flax spinners unlike cotton workers do not complain of the artificial humidity being harmful. In the summer of 1912, Dr T. M. Legge reported upon the body temperature of operatives in the wet spinning rooms and humid weaving sheds of linen mills. Temperature observations were taken of 31 males and 84 females. The temperatures were taken in the mouth shortly after commencing work and later on in the day: those of the men showed an average rise from 98°·4 F., normal, to 98°·8, while those of women rose from 98°·5 to 99°·2. When the wet bulb temperature reaches 75° F. the body heat of the workpeople invariably rises also. As regards elevation of temperature women exhibit a greater susceptibility than men.

The object of introducing moisture into flax spinning is to soften the gummy material in the flax fibre whereby its flexibility is increased and its tensile strength raised so that it can be drawn out and spun into finer yarn than is possible in the dry process. So complete is the ventilation that the temperature in a spinning room varies little between summer and winter. It is desirable that as regards the ventilation of linen mills, the present standard of 5 volumes of CO_2 per 10,000 in excess of that of the outside air should be maintained, special requirements being called for when the wet bulb temperature reaches 75° F., the point at which bodily discomfort begins. Should the wet bulb rise above 75° F., means should be taken to introduce 1000 cubic feet of air per hour for every linear foot of trough installed in the room. Artificial humidity should cease when the wet bulb reaches 80° F. The wet bulb temperature determines the degree of discomfort experienced by the workpeople. The nature of the employment and the amount of clothing worn are also of importance. When the wet bulb temperature reaches 88° to 90° F. the body temperature commences to rise even in persons stripped to the waist and doing no work. When once the temperature rises it may go on rising until symptoms of "heat stroke" appear unless the workman goes into the open air. Muscular work of itself raises the body temperature, hence the liability to "heat stroke" of soldiers in uniform on the march when the wet bulb temperature is only 70° F. Prolonged exposure to a hot moist atmosphere of a moderately high temperature is more injurious than exposure to a higher wet bulb temperature for a shorter period.

Apart from the effects of the work itself, too long hours spent at it are a cause of fatigue. This is especially true of work carried on by continuous processes. In some of the departments of steel and iron making, notably at the blast furnaces, the work goes on night and day; the fires are never extinguished for there are only two shifts per day of twelve hours each. Continuous work in the iron trade is said to be necessary owing to technical and economic requirements. If this was altered, work, we are told, would be disarranged, costs would be increased and a weekly restarting of the fires would entail considerable expense. Experience has shown that under certain circumstances, e.g. during a strike, blast furnaces can be damped down and be restarted fairly readily so that Sunday labour is not the absolute necessity it is stated to be, while the substitution of 3 shifts of men employed for 8 hours instead of 2 for 12 hours does not lessen but raises the wages of the men and at the same time improves their morale generally.

The good results which have followed the shortening of hours of work in the iron and steel industries of Great Britain have been equally observed in smelting works abroad. L. G. Fromont draws attention to two experiments carried out in the Works of the Société Anonyme des Produits Chimiques d'Engis, Belgium. Two decades ago the work was continuous in the smelting department. The men who looked after the furnaces worked a 24 hours' shift on end, lay off next day and night and recommenced work early on the following morning. Such sleep as the workmen might get during their idle day was interrupted by the men joining their family at meal times, so that all the sleep obtained would not be more than 10 to 12 out of the 48 hours. It was hardly to be wondered at therefore that the men were sometimes found asleep at their post by the night foremen, or that they sought in alcohol the stimulation necessary for their work. On leaving home in the early morning for the factory the wives and daughters used to give the men alcohol to take into the works, acting under the erroneous impression that alcohol sustained the men in their arduous labour and warded off fatigue. On returning home from the factory at 7.30 a.m., after 24 hours of continuous work, the men stopped at the public houses feeling the need of something to replace the energy they had lost during the long hours of continuous employment.

My own experience of some of the smelting works on the Continent enables me to corroborate what Fromont says, that both at Engis and elsewhere, in consequence of the hard work, long hours, deprivation of sleep and over-indulgence in alcohol, he found the men prematurely old and unfit for work. A 12 hours' shift was introduced at Engis with one 24 hours' shift every alternate Sunday. It was observed in the factory that during the hot months of summer the amount of zinc produced fell. The powers of the workmen declined to such an extent that the firm found it necessary to have relays of men ready to help those who had become fatigued and overcome by the heat. As the 12 hours' shifts were not followed by the results anticipated the firm resolved to give three 8 hours' shifts a trial—the men to work 8 hours with an interval of half an hour for food. It was arranged that each Sunday the men on the No. 2 shift should work 16 hours at a stretch so as to rearrange the shifts. At first the men resented the proposal but they gradually fell in with the new arrangements because not only was their period of rest per day increased, but instead of having to work every second Sunday a 24 hours' shift they had to work only every third Sunday, and then only for 16 hours instead of 24. The new method gave the workmen 35 full Sundays a year of complete rest instead of 26 with longer shifts. The effect upon the men has been that alcohol is no longer taken into the works and that drunkenness has disappeared. Sobriety, good behaviour and respect for cleanliness now mark the conduct of the men. The shorter hours of work have had an uplifting influence. Before they leave the factory the men wash themselves and change their clothes. Discipline has been more easily maintained, and greater cordiality exists between the men and their employers. The workmen's period of rest has been extended 36·8 per cent. The amount of material produced in the furnaces has increased 25 per cent. and in many instances although working a shorter shift, the men's wages have considerably improved.

Working overtime is another aspect of too long hours of work. In a large factory in the United States which I recently visited, and where work of a specialized character is carried on requiring careful and prolonged use of the eyes, the manager informed me that on occasions when the firm had been unusually busy the men had sometimes been asked to work overtime. When without leaving the factory one hour was added to the end of the day's work the additional results at first obtained began to dwindle after a few days. If the men left the factory at the usual hour, five o'clock, and returned after a meal at six o'clock and did two hours' work, not only was the production diminished after a few days, but so many mistakes occurred and so badly done was the work that in consequence of the amount of material spoiled and the reduction from wages which this entailed the firm found that it was not worth working overtime. Owing to the high class character of the work which the men had to do the strain upon the eyes was also more than they could bear.

As a cause of fatigue and of accidents mention must be made of imperfect illumination. Nothing surpasses sunlight and daylight. In factories in the United States the number of accidents is always greatest in the winter when artificial illumination has to be resorted to. Mr Leon Gaster, editor of *The Illuminating Engineer*, has shown how poor illumination of factories tends to diminish both the quality of work and the output. It neither pays the employer nor the employed. By the latter a severe strain is experienced, for the eyes have to be used more than they otherwise would be. Bad illumination means more spoiled work, a larger number of accidents and greater fatigue to workpeople. So far as eye strain is concerned it is not so much that the light is always deficient as that it is improperly distributed. During work the eyes should not be exposed to unshaded lights placed in the direct range of vision. Such lights create "a glare" which dazzles rather than illuminates. Light should fall upon the work a man is doing and not on his eyes. Reflected light from brightly polished metallic surfaces is equally objectionable. If lamps are used they should be completely screened from the eyes by suitable reflectors throwing the light where it is required. In factories where there is much dust floating in the atmosphere, the lamps should be cleaned frequently for, owing to the dust and dirt, much light is lost. Working with dark materials throws greater strain upon the eyes. Proper methods of lighting and distribution are absolutely essential. Where, for example, a man is working a machine the light should fall especially on the work.

Ocular fatigue arises from nerve conditions owing to the effort made by the individual to distinguish and fit in the details of his work—also by the image being too long retained upon the retina and creating an after-image. One of nature's methods of preventing fatigue consequent upon impressions made upon the retina is pupillary contraction. Too bright light should therefore be avoided just as much as defective light. In badly illuminated factories accidents are sure to occur. There should be no dark places where dangerous machinery is running. All flights of stairs should be well lighted, not by having a brilliant unshaded light at the top of the stairs, for a light placed there only dazzles the eyes and makes it difficult for persons to descend. It should be covered by a reflector and its surface so screened that the light is thrown down upon the stairs. Potteries and loco-motive works are frequently badly illuminated, so too are iron works, owing to the floor space being dull and covered with dark materials so that only from 2 to 3 per cent. of the incident light is reflected. From the molten metal too there is a glare which dazzles the eye and increases the risk of the men stumbling. It is therefore recommended that instead of having a few units of great concentrated brilliancy there should be a number of sources of moderate candle power placed fairly high up in the place where the work is carried on. The lighting of a factory is deemed to be insufficient if the illumina-tion taken on the horizontal plane, 1 foot above the floor, falls below one third of a foot candle.

Since many circumstances lead up to it we may well ask ourselves—What is fatigue? All work implies change and waste. In health, when work and muscular exercise are not carried too far, there follow a sense of satisfaction and a feeling of comfort and well being. Work when it exceeds the normal limit is followed by fatigue. Not only are the exercised muscles tired but there is a feeling of languor which suggests that the central nervous system has not escaped. Fatigue has therefore a local and a general significance. To the individual concerned, fatigue is an indication that he has reached his limitation, that expenditure has exceeded his energy producing powers and that his reserve is being called upon. The structural changes induced in nerve cells through work have been investigated by C. F. Hodges who found, on microscopically comparing the ganglionic nerve centres of bees before the morning flight with the same ganglia in other bees which had not been on the wing all day, that after a day's flight the nucleus and contents of the cells had undergone structural alterations which a night's rest and nourishment were capable of re-moving.

Fatigue has been the subject of study by many physiologists

whose opinions are collected and reviewed in an admirable book, *Fatigue and Efficiency*, by Miss Josephine Goldmark of New York. Unless fatigue or waste products are eliminated from the body they poison the nerve-endings in muscle, also the nerve cells of the brain, and thus become a source of danger. Sudden death has occurred in exhaustion owing to the large amount of toxin circulating in the blood. Hunted animals have died in the chase partly through fear and cardiac overstrain, partly also through poisoning caused by the retention of the chemical products arising from the wear and tear of the body. In fatigue, the blood becomes chemically altered: it becomes less alkaline. When the blood of a fatigued animal is injected into the veins of a healthy animal of the same species signs of fatigue are observed in the receiving animal. That the muscle substance is altered as the result of prolonged exertion, and that death may be the consequence of such exertion, are indicated by the readiness with which the muscles undergo putrefaction. In man it is rare for exhaustion to be followed by death, but it occurred in the case of Eukles of immortal memory, the runner from Marathon, who fell dead when announcing to his countrymen the victory by the Athenians over the Persians.

Professor Pierracini gives in detail the circumstances attending the death of two native runners in Algeria, one after covering a distance of 192 kilometres (120 miles) in 45 hours and the other 252 kilometres (156 miles) in 62 hours. In the body of each of these men abnormal rigidity developed and was followed by early putrefaction. From cases such as these where muscular exercise exceeded the limit of safety, it would appear that the chemical poisons or toxins which are generated within the individual are capable of destroying life. It is hardly necessary to allude to the excellent work done in this direction by the late Sir Michael Foster of Cambridge and Professor Mosso of Turin, the experiments by Professor Frederick S. Lee of Columbia University, also those of Professor Ranke, the German physiologist who demonstrated the development of fatigue by the injection into animals of fatigue products taken from a tired animal. When the blood becomes charged with waste products the central and peripheral nervous systems suffer.

Familiarity with toxins and antitoxins obliges us to raise the question, whether if fatigue is due to a toxin or toxins, there is no antitoxin available whereby fatigue can be averted? In 1904, Weichert, after having isolated from fatigued muscles a specific toxin which when injected into healthy animals caused fatigue, set himself the task of preparing an antitoxin which when administered in small doses would lead to the presence in the blood of a specific antitoxin whereby when the muscles of the animal are experimented upon they do not fatigue so readily as those of animals under ordinary circumstances. Experiments performed by other physiologists have not so far corroborated the opinions expressed by Weichert.

It is the experience of most of us that work done after fatigue has set in involves a corresponding greater expenditure of energy. Practically speaking what the individual feels under these circumstances can be demonstrated experimentally by stimulating fatigued muscles by means of electricity. Stronger and stronger stimuli are required until the time comes when the muscles cease to respond to any stimulus. Muscular work if graduated to a person's physical fitness and capacity improves the tone of muscle but if the exertion is prolonged there must be a period of rest commensurate with the amount of work done. That is one reason why we condemn the long hours, the 12 hours' shifts, which prevail in certain industries in which the processes of work are continuous.

In these days we find men and women of unequal powers of resistance crowded into factories and trying to keep pace with machinery. Sooner or later some of the workers become the victims of fatigue. Resistance to fatigue is not only a matter of health and physique but of sex as well. Woman is physiologically handicapped and therefore goes down more readily. Her sphere is narrower than that of man. The burden of industrial over-activity weighs more heavily upon her. The problem of fatigue becomes all the more important owing to the increasing number of young women who are forsaking home life for factory employment. Data concerning some aspects of fatigue problems are unobtainable because, notwithstanding what has been said, there are many women who are not only physically equal to men, who work as hard and who bear fatigue just as well as, if not better than, many men. This applies rather to the few than to most women. In cotton mills in Switzerland, where both sexes are employed, Schuler and Burckhard found the relative morbidity of men and women in the spinning department to be as 100 : 128, and in the weaving department 100 : 139. The duration of sickness among factory hands is higher for women than men. Even where the morbidity tables of Insurance Societies show men to be more frequently ill than women the duration of their sickness is shorter. Taking a Swiss Insurance Company I find, "among 100 insured men an average of 26·76 receive sick relief but among women only 24·26. The men who received sick relief averaged 23·55 days of illness, the women averaged 32·46." The women showed a lower percentage of relief but a longer average duration of sickness and as a result of these two circumstances the average morbidity of the women is higher than that of the men, 7·87 as against 6·30. In one of the German Insurance Societies for each 100 persons the men averaged 21·6 days lost through sickness and the women 24·4 days, while in an Austrian Society the men lost 16·5 days and the women 18·8. Generally speaking women lose more days from sickness than men: they are less able to bear the strain which modern industrial methods are imposing upon them.

Since Germany began to change from an agricultural to an industrial country there has appeared an increasing invalidity among her people. The increase in the amount of sickness is attributed to the harder and more exciting nature of the work. In 1902 in one district in Germany there were 487,000 persons invalided, in the same district in 1910 there were 893,585, an increase in the amount of sickness far in excess of the increase in the population.

Hard manual labour such as tilling of the soil, navvying, labouring in iron and steel works leads to structural alterations in the blood vessels of the workmen at an earlier date than the changes which are usually regarded as the result of age and of deranged metabolism. It is not uncommon to find workmen the subjects of a form of arterio-sclerosis although still comparatively young men. In the coal mines of Northumberland and Durham vascular changes do not show themselves until well after the age of 40, if at all, but I am told that in many of the coal mines of Fifeshire the miners are the subjects of structural alterations at an age quite a decade before this. On examining the thickened and degenerated walls of blood vessels of men who have worked hard, it would almost seem as if the physical strain they had been exposed to had been unequally distributed, for the pathological changes are more pronounced in the limbs which do the greatest amount of work, a circumstance which shows that there are other things in operation than toxins and waste products. Heredity also plays a part in the development of these pathological changes.

Coal mining is not only hard work but in order to win coal the men have to place themselves in awkward positions especially where the seams are narrow. The hours of work are 7 to 8 per day for $5\frac{1}{2}$ days one week, 5 the following week and this is repeated. It is difficult to say at what age a collier is at his best. When in consequence of the coal miners' strike in 1912 it was decided by the Government to introduce a minimum wage, it became necessary on the part of the miners themselves to admit that all the men were not physically equal, and that the output to some extent was influenced by the age of the miner. It was felt that whatever form legislation assumed work should not be taken entirely away from the older men, but that they should be given the opportunity of doing work at reduced wages.

I have tried to ascertain what is the period usually regarded in a miner's career as that in which he does his best work. There is a general opinion that this lies between the ages of 45 and 55. For a spurt a younger man may produce more but for steady work, endurance and average production over a length of time, the middle aged man is superior. Age imposes limitations, however, which cannot be ignored. To the influence of daily work must be added the cumulative effect of years of toil but, even allowing for this, age has yet claims for permission to work and which employers should not altogether disregard. In the United States speeding up of machinery and rushing are carried further than they are in this country with the result that there is employed in the factories a smaller percentage of elderly men than here. Except in a few arduous and badly paid occupations, "too old at forty" is not true. Physically, as already stated in regard to the working capacity of coal miners the best is yet to be after 40, while of men engaged in intellectual pursuits many achieve greater success and attain to greater heights in literature and art after the age of 40. It is equally true that ere the noonday of life is reached a man or woman has made a reputation to which succeeding work often contributes little if at all. Age like experience is personal. It is not simply a question of the number of years lived. One of the effects of recent legislation is that the older hands are being driven out of the factories. Employers believe that they incur greater liability by retaining the older workmen, but if age and experience are worth anything the influence of these should be apparent in the number of accidents at particular age periods. There is a feeling that older workmen are more careful. On the other hand their recoverability from sickness and accidents is slower. The liability to sickness is greater after 60 than before.

Whatever opinions we may hold in regard to hard work and advancing years, also the necessity of slackening off as the years go by, there can be only one opinion and that an adverse one, so far as concerns arduous work begun at too early an age, excessively long hours and the carrying of too heavy weights by boys and girls of tender years. Such things menace health, delay development, cause physical deformities and too frequently end in broken health. Legislation by raising the age at which work shall commence has removed some of the evils, but there are still to be found employers who impose upon young persons of both sexes physical burdens far beyond their strength.

What is true of children's work is also true of women's labour.

Sweated industries are unorganized. Owing to unregulated competition, the individual worker is left to secure the wages he or she best can, regardless of those obtained by others. Of men and women it is said that they work for their living. All of them however do not receive a "living wage." A "living wage" is not the same everywhere nor under all circumstances. It varies according to the education of the individual, his trade, and the locality in which the particular kind of work is carried on. It depends too upon nationality. It ought to be higher in large towns than in the country since house rents in towns are higher. The wages of a man are higher than those of a woman because it has been felt that the "man must receive sufficient to keep himself in a state of efficiency and at the same time to rear a family to a standard equal to his own." With the wages received, men and women ought to be able to purchase more than the mere necessaries of life. Unless these can be procured, the individual clearly is not receiving a "living wage." A woman is usually paid ⅓ to ½ of what a man receives, chiefly because hitherto women have been in the habit of accepting this as their due, and of taking the position as granted. The present war will probably alter some of these relationships. In a great many occupations the weekly wages fall short of the 21s. 8d. for married men, and of the 14s. to 16s. for single women which Mr B. S. Rowntree maintains is the lowest amount compatible with respectability. Not only are wages frequently insufficient to support life and to render it efficient, but the conditions under which the work is carried on are not always satisfactory from a health point of view. While it is in home industries that underpaid labour is principally found yet factory employment is not always free from this defect. The evil influence of small wages is intensified by inconstancy of employment.

In my visits to some of the sweated homes of Bethnal Green I have been struck by the long hours of work and the mere pittance received by the women. One, the mother of five children, I found making match boxes. By working from 7 a.m. till 9 or 10 p.m. she could make from 10s. to 11s. per week, out of which she had to pay 1s. for working expenses.

Another woman, a trouser finisher, received 2¼d. to 2½d. per pair of trousers, to finish which it took one hour and ten minutes. Her income was 9s. a week out of which she had to buy thread. A brush drawer, a widow 65 years of age, informed me that she could finish 6 brushes a day at the rate of 2¼d. each. She began this kind of work at the age of 6 years, and beyond the interruptions due to maternity she had been a brush drawer ever since. She pays 2s. 6d. a week for the one room in which she lives, works and sleeps. For "needle and thread" work, i.e. putting uppers on children's slippers women receive 7s. a week. Many of the women engaged in the home trades above mentioned, work 80 to 90 hours a week and make 7s. to 11s., an amount considerably below a "living wage."

Many of the sweated industries are connected with the ready-made clothing trades, but iron chain-making as carried on at Cradley Heath near Birmingham is, on account of the fatiguing nature of the work, one of the worst of all this class of industries. Women work in the chain-making industry from 7 a.m. till 8 p.m. or later and only receive 10s. a week— the girl apprentices 4s. Nail making, chain making, artificial flower making, dress and military uniform making, the making of safety-pins and of sacks, carding of hooks and eyes and buttons, with many others, are all included under sweated industries. All this type of home industry could be as well done, if not better, in a workshop or factory than in the homes of the people. To transfer the work to the factory would be doubtless to entail hardship upon many women who with children are so circumstanced that they could with difficulty leave their home for the factory. One strong objection to these home industries is the readiness with which the children of the family are drawn into the net of toil. If sweated industries are to be permitted, better terms must be arranged for the women. Want of union among female workers is one explanation of their helplessness in the matter of payment for work done. It is difficult to bring home-workers into line, whereby they can become organized so as to secure higher wages, and yet this has been done by the Anti-Sweating

League in the case of match box makers. The Trades Board
Act which was passed in 1909 arranges for the fixation of
minimum wages. Probably Trade Boards will in the future
play a helpful part in regulating the wages of home-workers.
In trades of even a complicated nature the fixing of a minimum
wage cannot present insuperable difficulties.

Despite insufficient feeding and the poverty of the surroundings of sweated workers, I found the women bright and
cheerful but, although I have no data to fall back upon,
my feeling is that the infantile mortality rate of the sweated
districts must be fairly high. Improper and insufficient feeding
destroys infant life, while anaemia with constipation and its
attendant evils is the bane of the young women workers. A
sweated mother, to whom every five minutes spent from work
is so much money lost, can ill afford the time to give her infant
the breast, to look after the other children as well, and to
keep the home attractive and tidy. Although the work is
sedentary, it is not of itself unhealthy: it is carried on in
small living rooms, many of which are so overcrowded with
goods that proper heating and ventilation become impossible.
The evils of sweating are the low rates of wages, excessive
hours of work and the unhygienic surroundings. Many of
the workers can only live by receiving poor law assistance.
Societies have been formed in the hope of remedying matters.
Of these the National Anti-Sweating League, the Women's
Co-operative Guild, and the Women's Trade Union League
are best known.

Artificial flower making

Artificial flowers are a luxury and not a necessity. It is
a city industry and Paris is its home, for in the French capital
the best flowers are still made. In the small workrooms in
Paris 16 per cent. of the artificial florists work less than 10
hours per day, 56 per cent. work from 10 to 12 hours, 28 per
cent. work from 12 to 16 hours and some of these occasionally
all night. Where it is a home industry the women work from
11 to 18 hours a day. Elderly workers whose eye-sight has

become enfeebled frequently commence work in the summer at 4 a.m.   While the home-workers outnumber those employed in the shops, 70 per cent. of them were found to have received their training in the shops.   Girls who learned the trade before their marriage follow it afterwards.   Child workers are few. This is owing to the high class character of the Parisian flowers and the requirement of skill.   Among the women, real artists are found: there are some who copy flowers brought from the gardens and who will spend 4 or 5 hours in making a rose.

In London, female artificial florists work 11 to 12 hours a day and receive 2½d. to 9d. per one dozen sprays, or about 9s. to 10s. per week.   As already indicated, owing to the higher class type of work, a Paris florist will make 4 to 5 francs or more per day, but the majority only 1 to 3 francs.   For small flowers such as violets, the wages in Paris are from 1 franc 5 cents to 2 francs per day.   Artificial flower making unfits women for other kinds of work.   The manner in which the nippers are held does not help the fingers to ply the needle, nor do the hands retain their suppleness and aptitude for house work.   There is only one other kind of work which goes well with artificial flower making and which may be taken up during the off-season and that is feather dressing. When the flower making season is over that for the dressing of feathers has come.   All artificial florists are not good feather dressers.   Feather dressing is an art by itself and has to be learned by apprenticeship.

I have seen something of artificial flower making both in this country and on the continent.   It is a poorly paid occupation as already stated, and like most of the sweated trades it is carried on in small and ill-ventilated rooms.   In Greater New York, in 1910, there were 7,292 women and 1,231 men employed in making artificial flowers.   In the United States the organization of the market has turned the art into a trade so that the work is carried on in workshops run by employers who sell the flowers by the gross.   The largest number of artificial florists are young women between the ages of 16 and 25.   According to the census, 55·3 per cent. of the women employed in artificial flower making earn less than 6 dollars (25 shillings) a week in the busy season and 25 per cent. earn less than 8 dollars (33s. 4d.). In the United States the flower making season begins in October and ends in May when the feather trade commences. A good deal of artificial flower making is done in the home. There, as in this country, the same objections hold: there is overcrowding, young children are pressed into the service at a time when they should be playing in the open air, the room is badly ventilated and home-work tends to cut down prices.

The work is nearly all done by the women sitting. 33 per cent. of the women who make the artificial French roses, especially the double roses, suffer in health through handling the flowers. They complain of headache, nasal catarrh, dryness of the throat probably from the dust, and also of vomiting. In at least one third of those who thus suffer the symptoms are those of metallic poisoning, for on examination of the red leaves of the roses several are found to contain salts of lead. The florists suffer too from pains in the arms and shoulders and their sight is early impaired by the bright colours of the flowers.

The women who follow this kind of work would make more out of their occupation if they were organized. It would be well for them if they served an apprenticeship and were taught artificial flower making artistically, for with flower making and feather dressing fashions change, and those women will alone be successful who can devise new colours and new groupings.

Before passing from the subject of artificial flowers I should like to draw attention to their effect upon the young women engaged in sale rooms, and where the flowers are collected and distributed. A few of them show a tendency to laryngeal and pulmonary catarrh attended by cough owing to the dust given off by the flowers. In the expectoration I have found on microscopical examination particles of dust identical with those given off from the flowers.

Feather cleaning

The feather industry is not free from risk. The feather sorters of the Eastern Province of South Africa are said not only to suffer from chronic bronchitis, but to exhibit a higher mortality from pulmonary phthisis than the population generally. Commencing with signs and symptoms of bronchitis the disease tends to gravitate into pulmonary tuberculosis. Dr W. Gilbert of Port Elizabeth Hospital has met with several cases of feather-sorters' phthisis. He is of the opinion that the malady commences as a broncho-pneumonia and is at first non-tuberculous. A subacute inflammatory affection of the nostrils is also met with. The cause of the illness is the dust shaken out of the feathers or the fluff. Steinhaus in an article on "Hygiene in the Bed Feather Industry," deals with the various methods of disinfecting feathers on a large scale, as in the feather cleaning works of Dortmund. Attention too is drawn by him to the possible risks which lurk in dirty feathers. He gives as an illustration the occurrence of an epidemic of small-pox in Breslau in 1906, and which was probably the result of infection introduced through uncleansed feathers from Russia. In the preliminary process of removing from feathers all such gross impurities as stones, animal excreta, and worms, also the finer dust removed by passing the feathers through revolving drums, a process which lasts for 10 minutes, he found that a sample of raw feathers from China lost 32 per cent. of their weight.

To cleanse feathers, after the preliminary methods just alluded to, they should be subjected to the action of steam under a pressure of 2½ atmospheres and a temperature of 137° C.: afterwards exposed to dry heat for 10 minutes and subsequently thrown into a room and allowed to settle. Severe as this treatment may appear it does not render the feathers bacteriologically sterile. To accomplish this it is necessary that during the process of steaming, formaldehyde should be added in the proportion of from 75 to 100 grammes per cubic metre of space of the disinfecting chamber.

Badly paid work is not always light work

Badly paid work is not always light work.   Three to four decades ago the horrors of the brick fields in England were made known to the public by George Smith of Coalville, so far as children's labour was concerned, but the strike of brick-workers in June, 1913, caused to be made widely known the hardships experienced by female brick-makers in the black country.   Girls from 16 to 18 years of age were found carrying loads of 2 cwt over a distance of 50 yards, working 10½ hours a day and making only from 6s. to 7s. a week.   Women were carrying loads of unbaked bricks at the rate of 2d. per ton, while others who shaped the bricks and whose wages were 11s. per week were handling the clay at the rate of 1d. per ton. The physical effects of this hard work accompanied by poor food, unhealthy home conditions and chronic fatigue, have already left their impress upon many of the workers as shown by the amount of spinal deformity which prevails.   We cannot wonder at the spinal column becoming crooked when girls 16 years of age are obliged to carry on their shoulders as much as 6½ tons of clay per day and for which they receive 14 pence.   Moulders, i.e. the women who make the bricks, receive 2s. 8d. to 3s. for 1000 bricks.   Standing in front of a bench a woman removes from the puddled mass in front of her a piece of clay sufficient in weight to make a 9 lb. brick, but to do this the mass lifted must weigh from 10 to 11 lb. The clay is banged into a mould and the superfluous clay scraped off.   The brick is then turned out on to a palette, and after the bricks have accumulated they are taken to the stove, placed on edge and left there all night.   Subsequently the bricks are stacked.   During this process a woman will lift 28 tons of bricks for which she receives 2s. 8d. or a little more than 1d. per ton.

In the brick fields the men work equally hard.   They pound the clay with naked feet into large moulds.   By the time these men reach the age of 40 they are old and crippled by rheumatism.   The men who empty the kilns are exposed to great heat: they perspire freely and become exhausted owing to lifting the heavy loads of bricks on to the shoulders of the girl carriers. Each man keeps six girl carriers pretty constantly on the track during the 10½ hours they are all employed. For this work, men receive 22s. to 23s. per week.

BIBLIOGRAPHY

Haegler, Dr Du. *Repos Hebdomadaire.* Estève de Bisch, Antwerp, 1907.
Goldmark, Miss Josephine. *Fatigue and Efficiency,* Parts I and II. Charities Public Committee, New York, 1912.
Cadbury, E. "Sweating." (Article by G. Shawn.)
Anti-Sweating League's Reports. 34, Mecklenburgh Square, London, W.C.
Bulletin du Ministère du Travail, Juin, 1913.
Kleek, Mary Van. *Artificial Flower Making.* New York Survey Associates, 1913.
Steinhaus. *Deutsche Vierteljahresschrift f. Öffentliche Gesundheitsflege,* Bd. 24 Heft (ii), 1912.
Seasonal Trades, by various writers, 1912. Constable and Co., London.
Smith, George. *The Cry of the Children from the Brick Fields of England.* Houghton, 1879.
Second Report of the Departmental Committee on Humidity and Ventilation in Cloth Weaving Sheds, 1911.
Report of the Departmental Committee on Humidity and Ventilation in Flax Mills and Linen Factories, 1914.
Report on Hours of Labour in Continuous Industries. International Association for Labour Legislation, 1912.
Fromont, L. G. *Une Expérience Industrielle de Réduction de la Journée de Travail.* Misch et Thron, Bruxelles, 1906.
Gaster, Leon. *Royal Institute of Public Health.* Congress of Paris, 1913.
Annual Report of the Chief Inspector of Factories and Workshops, 1912.
Hodges, C. F. *American Journal of Psychology,* 1887–1888, Vol. I, p. 479.
Pierracini, Prof. *Patalogia del Lavoro,* p. 18. Milan, 1906.
Weichert, W. "Über Ermüdungs toxine und deren antitoxine." *Münchener Med. Wochens.* 1904, 51, No. 1, p. 12.

CHAPTER IV

THE HEALTH AND COMFORT OF THE WORKER

FIRE ESCAPES IN FACTORIES. DRINKING WATER. LAVA-
TORIES AND BATH HOUSES. AIR SPACE. MESSROOMS.
SOCIAL WELFARE. AMBULANCE INSTRUCTION

It goes without saying that once workers are within a factory the employer is more or less responsible for their comfort and health. If this were not so the lives of employed persons would be endangered by work carried on in buildings structurally unsafe, hygienically unsound, and from which in the event of fire there might be practically speaking no escape. One of the requirements of factory construction is that there shall be

Fire escapes

In the United States the provision of fire escapes is carried to greater length than in Great Britain. Wherever more than 20 persons are employed in any place, several of the States demand that fire escapes shall be provided. Since each of the States of the American Union has its own laws, require- ment of fire escapes is not general. Where the law is enforced one of the results is an unseemly disfigurement of the buildings with these means of escape in emergency. Fire escapes may be simply towers of stone, brick, or cement situated at either end of a factory readily accessible from every part of the building, from each floor of the same and with ready egress to the ground. The stairs must be wide and fire proof. Instead of having the stairs enclosed there may be outside iron stairs descending all the way to the ground or to protected iron stations on the first floor, which when not required are cantilever gangways poised in the horizontal, but which immediately and gently become tilted when a person walking thereupon has proceeded beyond the centre of gravity of the gangways. By either of these means in the event of fire a factory can be fairly quickly emptied of its workers. The windows close to external fire escapes must be made of fire-proof glass so that there is small chance of the windows breaking and of flames issuing therefrom. In addition to such means of escape there should be as an annexe to each factory a water tower. Each factory should have its own fire brigade. Experience shows how undesirable it is that in factories there should be, unless in fire proof parts of the buildings, accumulations of waste inflammatory material. There should be no overcrowding beyond the limits of escape. The exits should be ample: there should be automatic water sprinklers in each room and smoking should be interdicted.

Even where all these means are provided they will not suffice in an emergency unless all the factory hands have been educated to the use of them. On the outbreak of a fire it is panic which does harm. By calmness tempered with discipline danger may be averted. Disorderly rushing to the vents of escape can be controlled by firmness and by the directions given by trained men in whom the work-people have confidence. All the men, women and girls should have fire drills every 2 or 3 weeks so that the workers, disciplined and controlled by the foremen of each floor, can be at once marshalled into order on the fire signal being sounded and proceed to the special exit of the floor and there await the word of command to descend.

In my recent visit to Trentham, U.S. America, I had the opportunity of witnessing fire drills with Colonel Bryant, Commissioner of Labour, New Jersey. Our visit to the first factory was unexpected. It was a large tobacco and cigar factory: the firm employed 1200 work-people. The means of escape were the ordinary inside wide stairs of two towers, one at either end of the factory. At the time the fire signal was rung all the hands were busily employed. In less than two minutes the women and girls were emerging from the stairways into the street in rows of four. Within three minutes the factory was completely emptied of all the workers, male and female. The procession of girls kept moving up and down the street in military order. Hardly had the male and female operatives emerged from the factory than the firemen were on the water tower ready, with hose in hand, to play upon the building. In some of the large factories when the fire alarm is sounded a similar message is sent to the local fire brigade of the town so that the engines are turned out immediately, and the town's firemen proceed also to the factory. In the State of New Jersey, law requires that new factories two storeys in height must have two means of egress from each floor—these may be inside stairways, outside fire escapes or both—also that all factories more than two storeys in height must have at least two means of egress, one of which shall be an inside stairway and one an outside fire escape or an approved tower, the means of egress to be increased as circumstances demand. Colonel Bryant is rather in favour of fire or stair towers than of fire escapes.

I also saw a large cotton mill in Trentham similarly emptied after the sound of the fire signal. It was a factory of five storeys. The women had to escape one by one down iron zig-zag stairs outside the factory. As the steps are rather steep, the stairs exposed, and only one worker could descend at a time, the women and girls, when at work, always wear an india-rubber band round their waist which in the event of the fire signal being sounded is at once pulled down over their skirt to near the knees so that during a high wind or otherwise, no embarrassment is likely to be created by displacement of the clothing during descent.

Drinking water

Next to good air if there is one thing required by people working in a high temperature it is a plentiful supply of pure drinking water. In every part of a factory facilities of obtaining pure water should be afforded. The water supply should be that of the town or of the district, and ought to come direct into the factory from the main. Factories in country districts should not make use of surface water lying close to the mills nor should stagnant water ever be introduced for drinking purposes. In ironworks where the men are exposed to great heat, water taps should be placed at frequent intervals in the sheds so that men can slake their thirst without being obliged to go some distance from their work. The old type of water tap with its iron mug on a chain has had its day. It is not desirable that drinking cups, out of which all can drink, should be used. There is always the risk of infection, besides it is not cleanly. In the steel works at Pittsburgh, U.S.A., I was struck by the simplicity of the water jet fountain, the purity and coolness of the water, also the cleanliness of the fountain generally. From the bottom of a metal basin there projects a small metal pipe through which when the water is turned on a jet of water is thrown upwards 14 or 15 inches, not with too great force, so that a workman gently inclining over the basin receives the jet of water into his mouth. There is no touching of any metal with the lips. In extremely hot weather means should be taken to cool the water supplied to men in the factory.

Lavatory convenience

Sanitary conveniences should be provided in sufficiently large numbers separately and disjointly for both sexes, readily accessible and in not too exposed or public part of a factory. Such places should be kept clean and in proper order by male and female attendants. In large iron works screened urinoirs should be so placed as to be readily reached by the men. It is monstrous to expect men when heated and perspiring freely, either during the day or night, to walk an unreasonable distance through the works, inside or outside, exposed to all kinds of weather to closets placed for example on the banks of a river simply for the convenience of the removal of the excreta. Men so employed should not be thus incidentally exposed to the risks of cold and rain. All sanitary conveniences in iron works should be close to the place where the men are working, be readily accessible, and urinoirs should be separate from water closets. Scrupulous cleanliness and repeated disinfection of these conveniences is a necessity, for when men are working hard and perspiring freely the urine

becomes concentrated. Repeated swilling of the urinoirs is
therefore desirable. The plans of a new factory should not
be passed unless they provide ample sanitary conveniences for
the work-people employed.

Washing accommodation

Should be ample. For men and women employed in dusty
trades the number of washhand basins should be greater
than in trades which are not dusty. Soap and towels should
be provided by the employers. Each worker should receive
a clean towel at least once a week, washed at the expense of
the employer and he should have his own peg upon which to
hang it. There should be wardrobe accommodation close
to the washing room where the clothes can be kept. Each
worker should also have a locker and be given a key for it.

Bath houses

In all factories and workshops where the occupation is of
a dusty or dangerous nature, or where Home Office Regulations
require that a bath shall be taken, there ought to be bath
houses separate from the main building, heated and with a
sufficient number of bath rooms or cubicles supplied with hot
and cold water and so screened by curtains that the bath can
be taken with comfort. At one of the large collieries in
Westphalia which I visited, also at Brigue and Iselle during
the tunnelling of the Simplon I found the clothes rooms lofty
and well warmed. In these rooms the workman left the
clothes in which he worked and next morning he would find
them dried and comfortable to put on. I am not in favour
of one common spray room in which men and boys wash
together. This is a weakness of the Continental system. In
the cubicle and private bath rooms there should be spray or
shower baths as well. Attendants should see that the bath
and change rooms are kept warm and clean and that decorum
is maintained. Everything should be done by employers to
encourage cleanliness and to raise the self-respect of the
workers. This cannot be done if, as I have seen in some

British factories, workmen are expected to take a spray bath in a dark corner partitioned off from the workroom and about the size of a sentry box and wherein neither daylight nor artificial light is available.

Opinions differ as to whether coal miners should have their bath at the pit head at the end of their shift or in their own home. The homes of the British coal miners are small: they have no bath room; the accommodation is extremely limited, especially if there is a family of children. Miners have frequently a considerable distance to walk from the pit mouth to their home: they carry by their clothes and their boots mine dust and dirt into the home. Where wash houses are provided at the mouth of the pit the miner has his warm bath and is refreshed, he exchanges his wet and dirty clothing for his ordinary wearing apparel, he goes home with a better appetite than, when begrimed with dust, he has yet his tub before him.

Money would be well spent by colliery proprietors if they gave the miners better and ampler housing accommodation. There is too little consideration shown in this respect to men with large families. Mine owners should be as much opposed to overcrowding as hygienists and they ought to have practical knowledge of the conditions under which individually their work-people are housed.

Air space

In humid textile factories other than those in which cotton cloth is made, 600 cubic feet of fresh air per hour per person was the standard in 1902. This was a considerable advance upon the 250 cubic feet per head required by the Act of 1895. The legal limit at present is one of 12 volumes of CO_2, i.e. carbonic acid, per 10,000 volumes of air, but in foggy weather it is difficult to enforce this standard. In the winter when artificial lighting by gas and oil is called for, the production must not exceed 20 volumes of CO_2 per 10,000. Where in a workroom the amount of CO_2 equals 6 per 10,000 volumes of air, that room to any person entering it feels "close." The quantity of CO_2 present in the air is generally taken as the basis of ventilation. Although regarded as a measure of impurity of the air, CO_2 is no longer considered the deadly gas it was formerly believed to be. Every attention given to the health of the employees is in the end a financial gain to the employer so that in one sense the conditions under which work is carried on have something to do with the profits which are made.

The importance of ventilation can be seen from the statement supplied by Dr C. E. A. Winslow of what occurred in the New England Telephone and Telegraph Company at Cambridge, Mass., U.S.A. An improved ventilating system was introduced into the operating room in the spring of 1907. At first the change in the ventilation did not affect the attendance in the operating room during the summer of 1907 because, at this time of the year, the windows are open and ventilation is generally good. The improvement began with the winter months of 1907–1908. "For the first three months of 1906 the average percentages of operators absent were 4·9, 5·6 and 4·1 respectively: for 1907 the figures were 5·2, 5·0 and 3·4: for 1908 these dropped to 1·8, 2·4 and 1·5. Comparing the three winter months only (Jan., Feb., March) it appears that 4·9 per cent. of the force were absent in 1906, 4·5 per cent. in 1907 and only 1·9 in 1908. This means a net saving of 2·8 per cent. of the force employed corresponding to $1\frac{8}{10}$ of the entire time of one operator."

Mess rooms

Should be provided for those workers whose home is too far from the factory for them to travel for the midday meal. The transformation of any disused room in a factory into a dining room without regard to its situation, comfort and internal decoration is hardly the desirable way of meeting requirements. In the canteens of some of the large factories in the United States stimulants used to be sold, but where this permission has been withdrawn and only the sale of non-alcoholic drinks allowed there has been a distinct reduction in the number of casualties.

Social welfare

With few exceptions, such as for example at Cadbury's and the works of Messrs Lever Bros., little has been done in Great Britain in the way of social welfare by employers for the workers. I have had the opportunity of seeing what has been done in this direction in the United States by the Shredded Wheat Company at Niagara Falls and by other large firms. There, the mess rooms are ample, light, clean and are well furnished. Meals are sold at a cheap rate and served in an attractive manner, so that the midday meal makes a pleasant break in the day's work. For persons with weak digestion special meals are arranged. There are sitting rooms for both sexes to which the workers can retire after a meal. Here are found the daily papers and magazines, here too is a piano. When the weather is fine the employees in the dinner hour can go into the grounds, or they can go to the roof garden from which a splendid view of Niagara river and the surrounding country can be obtained. There are also rooms, with 1–3 beds, to which a girl can be removed if taken ill at work, and where there is always a nurse in charge. There is a large room for concerts, theatrical performances, social re-unions and balls during the winter months.

I admit that the Shredded Wheat Company's works are rather a show place, and that the cleanly character of the industry lends itself to its being such, but in other cities in the United States and in occupations of not so cleanly a nature I found similar arrangements prevailed. There is not the least doubt that the social welfare of the workers has not received in our country the attention it has received on the other side of the Atlantic. Dining rooms, reading rooms and meeting rooms are provided in many British factories for the employees, but excepting in two or three instances they have nothing of the brightness, attractiveness and cleanliness of those seen in France, Germany and the United States.

Ambulance instruction—First Aid

In mines, iron and steel works and in all factories where many hands are employed there should be an ambulance corps of men and women, trained to render first aid in case of accident and to deal within limits with emergencies. The advantages to the workers of this early assistance are beyond all question, especially as seen in the immediate and aseptic treatment of wounds. Too many of the minor wounds of working men become septic. Death has followed trivial injuries. No injury in a factory followed by an open wound, however insignificant, should be ignored. It makes all the difference to the workman if his wounds are at once cleansed and treated antiseptically. At collieries where immediate antiseptic treatment of wounds has been given effect to, the duration of incapacity for work has been diminished by from 2–3 days. The saving of health and of the men's time makes ambulance work a necessity. Shipyards must now, according to Home Office Regulations, be provided with stretchers, also surgical dressings kept in a convenient and accessible place, and they must have men trained in ambulance work.

In large iron works, at collieries and in large textile factories there should be a small hospital with 2–3 beds. At one of the collieries close to Newcastle there is such a building. It has to my knowledge served a useful end, and been the means of averting much suffering, if not of saving life. Men who have been seriously injured in the pit can be taken to the hospital adjoining the mine and be treated there or be allowed to rest and recover from shock before being taken by an ambulance to the Newcastle-upon-Tyne Infirmary.   Minor cases can be operated upon in the small hospital and recovery thus made more assured. Chloroform and Listerism have transformed surgery and have robbed operations of much of their horror. But for these our industrial fatalities would be greater.

CHAPTER V

OCCUPATION AND AGE FITNESS.   OCCUPATION AND MORTALITY

It has been shown by Dr John Tatham and other Statisticians that the mortality of men employed in various occupations is seriously affected by the surroundings in which the men work, and that these surroundings vary for the same occupation in different parts of the country. Tatham divides England and Wales into *Industrial Districts*. The County of Lancashire is taken as the seat of the cotton industry: the towns of Huddersfield, Halifax and Bradford as the seat of the woollen industry: Wolverhampton, Birmingham, Leeds and Sheffield as that of iron and steel, and Leicester as the seat of the manufacture of boots and hosiery. In the *Agricultural group* are included all the counties of England and Wales in which at least one-third of the occupied males over 10 years of age were returned at the last census as farmers and farm labourers. In order to compare the mortality among coal miners, statistics are taken from six local areas: (1) Durham and Northumberland, (2) Lancashire, (3) the West Riding of Yorkshire, (4) Derbyshire, (5) Staffordshire and (6) Monmouthshire with South Wales. Dr Tatham's figures deal with males 15 years of age and upwards.

The mortality in a given industry at any particular time can only be regarded as a rough measure of the healthfulness of that industry. Some occupations are simply unhealthy, others are positively destructive to human life. Occupation therefore is not always the source of health it ought to be. Coal mining and railway work are not unhealthy, but in following their calling the men are exposed to the risk of accidents, whereas in steel grinding, file cutting and the manufacture of white lead the risk to health from the occupation itself is the notable feature. It is not easy to assign to particular trades their influence for harm upon the work-people who follow them, for in unskilled trades the men keep changing their occupation. No matter what the occupation may be there are circumstances in the lives and habits of the work-people themselves which must be considered as tending to raise the mortality rate. Of these, intemperance in the use of alcohol, casual employment and poverty, also the rush of work during busy seasons, tend to increase the mortality rate of an occupation.

The greater use and application of machinery enable men and women less physically developed than their forebears to undertake work which but for machinery would not be possible. Machinery is reacting upon the men and women of to-day and is evolving a quick and alert class of worker upon whose highly-strung nervous system is being imposed special burdens created by the strain and fatigue of hours of constant watchfulness. Are the modern men and women really overworked in this age of stress and hurry? and if so at what age ought they to retire? "Too old at forty" was never seriously meant by Sir William Osler for physicians, literary men, Members of Parliament, prime ministers and the heads of large commercial houses. These men are only coming to their best after the age of 40. In the present war with Germany the ages of the commanders of the Allies is for each beyond 60 and at the time of writing there is nothing to show that Sir John French and General Joffre are less capable of enduring the strain of the campaign than the younger officers. We do not count age by years. It is the individual himself and the life he has lived that we think of. It must be admitted that there are occupations characterized by hard manual labour, in the following of which through exposure to inclement weather the men become prematurely old. Many boilersmiths and iron workers are old at 60.

To all of us there inevitably comes a time when it is necessary to lower the sail and haul in the rope, but the age at which this becomes necessary is not the same for all men even in the same occupation. It is the personal element in all men which should determine the age of retirement from active work and not the number of years lived. After man's entry into the sixth decade there is in most men a loss of elasticity and resiliency, but the work turned out by the sexagenarian and the regularity of his attendance in the office and in the factory compare most favourably with those of men who have only reached the forties. Circumstances however have arisen in connection with recent legislation for coal miners which have necessitated the assignment of values to age-periods based upon production, since owing to the hard work of the coal miner it is known that as age advances the producing power of the individual falls.

As already stated, p. 36, not only is coal getting hard work, but the work is carried on occasionally in awkward positions for the body. Fortunately the hours are shorter than in most occupations. When the House of Commons recently had under consideration a minimum wage for coal miners the men themselves had to admit that output was influenced by age. By this admission the Bill was so framed that the older men did not lose their employment. They are therefore allowed to work at reduced wages. The age of 57 was fixed upon as that for miners who were in constant employment. This is the age up to which the minimum wage can be claimed. For day workers or "datals" the age was fixed at 63. It had been found that older men could not produce coal to the same amount as their juniors. In discussing this subject with Mr William Straker of the Northumberland Miners' Conciliation Board so as to ascertain what the trade itself regards as the best period of a miner's life, from a strenuous point of view, he gave me the period of 45 to 55 as that during which men do their best work. For a spurt the younger man may produce more, but for steady work, endurance, and average production over a length of time, the middle-aged man is the superior.

Of all occupations that of the farmer is the healthiest. Close upon the farmer comes the clergyman. The agricultural classes spend much of their time in the open air. Anxious as they of necessity are on the approach of the harvest as to the state of the weather, farmers are on the whole less worried than persons in trade and commerce. The life of the average

clergyman is not regarded as an arduous one.   During the last
four decades, conditions of labour all round have been improving
and in consequence of this and industrial legislation the number
of deaths in certain trades has fallen.   Dusty trades still show
too high a mortality, but they are receiving the attention of
the Home Office. Apart from maladies caused directly or
indirectly by poisoning, such as that due to lead or arsenic,
the high mortality rate in most occupations, especially those
of a dusty nature, is due to diseases of lungs and tuberculosis.
It is not maintained that respiratory diseases and pulmonary
tuberculosis are the result of occupation alone, for there are
frequently contributory causes operating which are not always
easy of elimination.   The fact remains however that inhalation
of dust is the main cause of the ill-health of persons following
certain trades also of their high mortality.   These are shown in
the accompanying table (p. 59) taken from Dr John Tatham's
article "Dust-Producing Occupations."

From this table it will be seen that there are twenty
"industries in each of which the mortality from tubercular
phthisis and respiratory diseases together is more than double
that of agriculturists."   In some of the occupations the total
mortality from these diseases ranges from three times, to as
much as four and a half times that of the agricultural class.
A glance at the second column shows how dangerous some trades
are compared with others.   The manufacture of pottery and
earthenware occupies an unenviable position.   In some of the
branches of manufacture the workers are exposed to two
dangers, clay dust as affecting the lungs and lead dust from the
dried glaze which induces plumbism.   Potters are an unhealthy
class; they are especially prone to phthisis, to diseases of the
respiratory system and heart affections.   While they exhibit
a high death rate from phthisis their mortality rate from
bronchitis is four times as high as that of occupied males in
the aggregate.   Much of the phthisis from which potters die
is of a non-tuberculous type especially at its inception.   In
a similar manner in consequence of the character of the dust
which is inhaled, cutlers and scissor makers have a high
mortality from diseases of the lung and from phthisis.   High

in all age-periods the mortality figure beyond the 35th year " exceeds the standard among occupied males generally by from 64 to 72 per cent."

Comparative Mortality from Specified Causes in certain Dusty Occupations

Occupation	Comparative mortality figure (all causes)	Phthisis and diseases of respiratory system		Mortality figure		
		Mortality figure	Ratio	Phthisis	Diseases of respiratory system	Diseases of circulatory system
Agriculturist ...	**602**	**221**	**100**	**106**	**115**	**83**
Potter, Earthenware manufacturer	1702	1001	453	333	668	227
Cutler	1516	900	407	382	518	167
File maker ...	1810	825	373	402	423	204
Glass maker ...	1487	740	335	295	445	157
Copper worker ...	1381	700	317	294	406	186
Iron and steel manufacturer	1301	645	292	195	450	162
Zinc worker ...	1198	587	266	240	347	126
Stone quarrier ...	1176	576	261	269	307	137
Brass worker ...	1088	552	250	279	273	126
Chimney sweep	1311	551	249	260	291	142
Lead worker ...	1783	545	247	148	397	272
Cotton manufacturer	1141	540	244	202	338	152
Cooper and wood turner... ...	1088	526	238	250	276	137
Bricklayer, mason	1001	476	215	225	251	130
Tin worker ...	994	451	204	217	234	124
Wool manufacturer	991	447	202	191	256	131
Locksmith ...	925	428	194	223	205	104
Blacksmith ...	914	392	177	159	233	136
Baker—confectioner ...	920	392	177	185	207	130

One of the most unhealthy occupations is file cutting. The death rate from all causes is in this trade three times as high as that of agriculturists. Dust and lead are the causes which contribute to the high mortality. Of all persons working among metals and metallic dust, lead workers stand out badly. Although not *per se* a large industry yet many persons are brought into contact with lead directly and indirectly that the part which lead plays in the arts and manufactures becomes extremely important. Tatham found in one hundred occupations no fewer than thirteen in which lead poisoning became possible, and he gives the following as representing the comparative mortality figures from lead poisoning in certain trades:

Lead worker ...	...	211	Coach maker	...	7
File maker	...	75	Gasfitter, locksmith ...		6
Plumber	...	21	Lead maker ...	...	5
Painter and glazier ...		18	Printer	... ...	3
Potter ...	...	17	Cutler	... ...	3
Glass maker ...	...	12	Wool manufacturer ...		3
Copper worker	...	8	Occupied males	...	1

While these figures show the comparative mortality rates from lead poisoning in several trades it is not always easy to gauge the *relative damage* sustained by operatives as a result of their occupation. Lead workers for example are all more or less brought into contact with lead, whereas in the manufacture of earthenware it is principally the dippers, dippers' cleaners and glost placers who are thus circumstanced, so that while only one-twelfth of potters are brought into contact with lead, the deaths from lead poisoning are distributed over the whole body of potters and thus a false impression is created as to the amount of harm done by lead in the manufacture of pottery and earthenware.

Leaving metal workers, whom I shall discuss later, space will only permit of a few occupations being mentioned here. Others will be dealt with subsequently. Workers in textile factories show a high death rate from phthisis and diseases of the respiratory system. They are also prone to acute rheumatism.

The dangers of foul air although less than those due to dust are yet considerable as the following table also taken from Tatham's article shows:

Comparative Mortality from several causes in certain unhealthy occupations.

Occupation	Comparative mortality figure (all causes)	Phthisis and diseases of the respiratory organs		Mortality figure		
		Mortality figure	Ratio	Phthisis	Respiratory diseases	Circulatory diseases
Agriculturists	**602**	**221**	**100**	**106**	**115**	**83**
Bookbinder	1060	543	246	325	218	115
Printer	1096	540	244	326	214	133
Musician	1214	522	236	322	200	191
Hatter	1109	511	231	301	210	141
Hairdresser ...	1099	489	221	276	213	179
Tailor	989	466	211	271	195	121
Draper	1014	441	200	260	181	135
Shoemaker ...	920	437	198	256	181	121

Work carried on in ill-ventilated rooms the air of which is rendered impure by stoves and artificial illuminants, also sedentary occupations, predispose to phthisis and to diseases of the respiratory organs. In the order of mortality from these diseases the occupations are tabulated as to render the point at once apparent that the combined mortality from phthisis and respiratory diseases varies from twice to two and a half times that of agriculturists.

As regards the mining industry I find that according to the census of England and Wales 1911 there were employed of males above the age of 10 years the following: 503,294 as coal and shale workers, 278,924 workers below ground at the face, and 102,312 workers above ground, giving a total of 884,530. In iron mines there were employed 22,299 men, in tin mines 7125 and in lead mines 2968. The bulk of those enumerated above spend a considerable part of the day underground. Coal mines are well ventilated owing to the double shaft required by law and the pumping in of air. Except at the face, coal miners work in good air. This is not quite the case as applied to several of the lead mines. Coal mines vary in temperature according to their depth. Some of them are damp. Coal mining is not such an unhealthy occupation as at first sight it might appear. In the following table the mortality figures in each column represent proportions of the standard figure, the latter taken in each case as 100:

Occupation	Years of age						
	15—	20—	25—	35—	45—	55—	65 and upwards
Occupied males	100	100	100	100	100	100	100
Mining Industry	**148**	**112**	**87**	**78**	**95**	**121**	**147**
Coal miner	150	111	86	77	94	119	143
Durham and Northumberland	154	111	75	66	79	97	152
Lancashire	163	107	88	94	110	140	150
West Riding	115	92	76	77	89	126	138
Derby and Notts ...	93	68	69	59	73	96	118
Staffordshire	95	109	82	70	95	135	180
Monmouth and Wales...	227	141	118	97	117	140	129
Ironstone miner	134	90	82	66	83	91	144
Copper miner...	—	158	129	146	118	127	170
Tin miner	116	139	111	115	161	180	178
Lead miner	118	127	130	109	116	182	240
Mine service	127	264	129	98	95	113	155

(The bracket at left labels "Coal miners" spanning the Durham through Monmouth rows.)

Tatham's figures are based upon the census of 1891, when the number of persons employed was not so large as in 1911, but the facts remain in proportion much the same. "From the ages of 15–20 and from 20–25 as well as at both the age-groups above 55 years, miners in the aggregate die more rapidly than do other occupied males, whilst at intervening ages they die less rapidly." Coal getting is strenuous work. The men who follow the occupation are usually a hardy and well-developed class, although after having worked for years their knees give way and their legs become weak owing to the cramped position they are obliged to remain in, also the strain upon their knees. That coal mining is a risky occupation is shown by the high mortality from accidents. Tatham has eliminated the influence of "accident" and gives the following table to show the comparative mortality of the various groups of miners: (1) from all causes except accident, (2) from accident or violence, and (3) from disease and accident together.

Occupation		All causes except accident	Alcoholism	Liver diseases	Phthisis	Respiratory diseases	Bright's disease	Accident	Disease and accident together
Mining Industry... ...		**800**	**4**	**18**	**109**	**267**	**19**	**135**	**935**
Coal miners		784	4	17	97	269	18	141	925
Coal miners	Durham and Northumberland	678	5	23	94	156	15	96	774
	Lancashire	914	5	17	102	389	17	155	1069
	West Riding	798	4	16	123	288	16	114	912
	Derby and Notts ...	638	2	18	69	159	8	89	727
	Staffordshire	817	2	8	83	319	22	135	952
	Monmouth and Wales	902	7	16	107	345	27	243	1145
Ironstone miners		688	4	20	90	204	15	86	774
Copper miners		1195	—	28	331	347	68	35	1230
Tin miners		1361	4	28	508	377	29	48	1409
Lead miners		1267	5	34	380	325	33	43	1310
Mine service		946	6	42	114	216	20	75	1021
Farm labourer		590	4	13	115	129	12	42	632
Occupied males		897	13	27	185	221	27	56	953

Miners are not an intemperate class of men basing this statement upon the numbers who die from alcoholism. Their accident mortality rate is high in the early years. When this is deducted the industry shows a good record. The difference in the mortality rate in the various coal fields is interesting and is not readily explained. It may be due to the depth of the mines, their geological constitution, temperature and dampness. Phthisis is less frequent among coal miners than might be expected, but their death rate from non-tuberculous lung diseases is high. Their mortality rate due to phthisis is only about one-half of what it is in occupied males, but their mortality from respiratory diseases is greater by 21 per cent. Ironstone mining is a declining industry in this country. Tin mining is an unhealthy occupation. It shows high mortality figures for phthisis and respiratory diseases.

The working and the leisured classes

The mortality figures for *occupied* and *unoccupied* males carry a lesson. Between 25 and 65 years of age the figures are 953 and 2215 respectively. "In other words, the number of males of definite age constitution, within these limits, that would give 1000 deaths among the general population, and 679 deaths in the healthy districts, would give 953 deaths among occupied, and 2215 among unoccupied males. The comparative figure of unoccupied males, therefore exceeds that of occupied males by 132 per cent." Nearly two-thirds of the excessive mortality of unoccupied males as compared with occupied is due to either diseases of the nervous system or to phthisis.

BIBLIOGRAPHY

Tatham, John, M.D. Articles in *Dangerous Trades* (Oliver), pp. 135, 142, 149, 156. Also Decennial Supplement to 55th Report of the Registrar General, Vol. II.

CHAPTER VI

CHOICE OF A CAREER—BOYS AND GIRLS. FEMALE LABOUR. FEMALE SICKNESS RATES COMPARED WITH THOSE OF MALES

The choice of occupation by a boy is in many instances haphazard since a trade is frequently forced upon a youth owing to the financial requirements of his home at the particular time. Occupations too are taken up and dropped. Some persons fall into commercial and industrial positions more or less accidentally. The future of a boy on leaving school is less discussed by and talked over with the schoolmaster in this country than it is in Germany. In Germany the medical officer to the school examines the boys who are leaving so that those who are found to have weak lungs are advised not to

take up a sedentary but an outdoor occupation. It makes all
the difference as regards the future of a boy and girl if they are
allowed to choose their own occupation, since neither will be
happy unless employed in work which is congenial to him or to
her. On the other hand there is no reason why the advantages
and disadvantages of certain trades should not be placed by
a schoolmaster before the senior pupils. To what extent this
treatment of the subject would lessen caprice and alter personal
inclination it is impossible to say. In colliery districts the
choice of occupation is largely a matter of heredity. The male
members of a miner's family hardly look to any other occupation than that of the mine because the wages of pit boys are
good, the lads can remain at home and for a period the
parents benefit by the earnings of their sons. The daughters
of coal miners remain at home or go into domestic service.

Coal mining and such laborious occupations as navvying,
blast furnace work, boilermaking and engine-fitting can only
be undertaken by men of good physique. It is only strong
lads who can take up such work. Nearly all the men who
have drifted into these occupations are more or less selected,
but the widespread use of machinery has created a class of
artisan who is less physically developed than his predecessors.
Events in the present war however have shown that there is
nothing of the physical deterioration of the British race which
had been suspected. If we are in search of strong, powerfully
built, well-developed muscular men the best types are to be
found among men working as navvies or as labourers at the
blast furnaces in iron works. Many of them are Irish. The
excessive physical demands made upon those who follow such
occupations oblige many of them to fall out of the ranks as
the years roll on and to seek less arduous employment.

The sickness and mortality rates in a given industry are
a rough measure of the healthfulness of that industry at the
particular period. Most occupations are healthy, a few are
unhealthy and fewer still are positively harmful. There are
certain occupations, for example coal mining and railway work,
which are not of themselves unhealthy but in which the risk
to life is great through accident: there are others such as file-

cutting and steel grinding, also the manufacture of white lead in which the risk to health is a noteworthy feature. It is not always easy to assign to particular industries the influence for harm upon those who follow them, for in unskilled trades workmen as already stated elsewhere in these pages keep changing their employment. No matter what the occupation is, there are circumstances in the lives and habits of the work-people themselves which tend to raise the mortality rate. Of these, alcohol, casual employment, fairly constant work in dangerous processes, and the rush of work in busy seasons, are some of the circumstances which raise the sickness and mortality rate of a particular trade without necessarily being special to it.

Reverting to the question of choice of occupation by young adults the two main points which should help towards a decision are physical health and education. The former allows of certain occupations only being entered upon, while deficiency of education disqualifies for others. Accident of birth and social position at this part of our enquiry can be set aside. Fathers of poor parentage, but who have risen in the world, keep pointing out to their children the advantage of education and they seek to supply a better one than they themselves received. The extent to which education has been taken advantage of and the inclinations and wishes of youths are some of the guiding elements in coming to a decision. The question resolves itself into whether it shall be skilled or unskilled labour. One occupation always open to boys and girls leaving school at the earliest age is that of messenger. The work of a telegraph boy is an illustration. Dead-end trades which lead to nothing are never so satisfactory as those in which youths may rise to higher positions. Boys who have received a good average education should choose as far as they can a skilled trade. Although in unskilled labour the wages for boys may at first be good, yet as manhood is reached the wages do not rise in proportion and when bad times come the unskilled labourer is the first to suffer. Boys should choose a trade which is in the ascendancy and not on the decline, one too in which risk to health and life from accident or from other causes is small.

The choice of occupation has been widened in recent years by the increasing extent to which electricity is being used in the arts and sciences, also for illumination and transport. There is a tendency to underrate from a social point of view all work done by the hands as against that done by the brain. There is a feeling, for example, because a boy, the son of a working man has taken on the advantages of education as seen in his hand-writing and arithmetic, that such a youth should seek a more refined occupation than that of his father. The result of this has been that there are more clerks than are always necessary. The supply being greater than the demand salaries have kept low in consequence. A few clerks it is true ultimately attain high positions. They may become partners in, or the head of, the firm they entered as office boys, but the majority have to content themselves with salaries sometimes less than that of artisans in highly skilled trades. To young men endowed with inventive ability and who are neat-handed craftsmen, factory life supplies opportunities for unlimited development. It is given only to few to take advantage of the opportunities.

On the part of girls there is a growing tendency for them to enter shops, offices and factories than to stay at home or enter domestic service. After twenty years have been spent in any of these capacities it will be found that the average woman who chose domestic service is if she has been thrifty probably as well off financially as, if not better than, her sisters who went into a factory. She may not have had the same freedom and opportunity of spending her evenings, Saturday afternoons and Sundays as she pleased, but the fact of having had fewer abstractions has enabled her to save more from her wages and at the same time she has all along been qualifying herself for those duties which most women fortunately still regard as their true avocation, the head of a home. Domestic service which is the legitimate calling of most women should be made more attractive than it is by employers giving higher wages, greater opportunities for rest and leisure and by providing better sleeping accommodation. With the extended opportunities of learning housewifery at school, more girls should take to cooking as a career. Cooks are always required, they command high wages and if they marry, their experience has always a money value.

Office work, type writing and shorthand offer attractions to many girls. The work is clean and if carried on in light, well-ventilated offices it is healthy. One objection to it is its sedentary nature and the fact that it involves too much sitting and too little exercise. Teaching in schools has many advantages: although the work is trying the hours are not long and holidays are frequent and ample. The telephone has given a new occupation to women, but by highly-strung girls of an excitable nature and whose nervous system is likely to break down under strain it ought to be avoided. In the United States of America, Dr Emory R. Hayhurst found a high death rate from pulmonary consumption among female telegraph and telephone operatives. This is not our experience in Great Britain. In the State of Ohio women clerks, female book-keepers and stenographers head the list of all occupations as regards shortness of life. He gives the following as the percentages of persons dying from tuberculosis in the under-mentioned occupations: female boot and shoe operatives 31·8; female clerks and copyists 31·9; female bookkeepers and accountants 35·7; male stenographers and type writers 37; female stenographers and type writers 38·8; female cigar and tobacco operatives 40·3, and female telegraph and telephone operatives 43 per cent.

Statistics show a difference in the mortality rates between male and female workers. Generally speaking it may be said that when women have to earn their own living they exhibit a higher sick rate than men engaged in the same trade. British statistics supply less information on this point than German. In Stettin, 1902 to 1903, also 1908 to 1909, the sick rates in the case of male teachers were 2·8 and 5 respectively; for female teachers they were 6·4 and 10·3: as regards days lost through sickness during 1904 and 1905, also 1908 and 1909, male teachers lost 6·7 days and female teachers 14·8.

Prinsing found when both sexes are employed in the same

occupation that females have a higher sick rate than males. Between the ages of 15 and 60 he found:

	Males	Females
Tailors	56	61
Bookbinders	60	80
Brick and cement works ...	101	91
Textile trades	80	92
Clothing trades	86	96
Pottery and porcelain works ...	93	105

The Leipzig Insurance Fund supplies the following per 100 persons employed generally:

	Cases of sickness with inability to work, percentage	Days of sickness
Male insured persons	39·6	855
Female insured persons ...	41·8	1030
Male not insured persons ...	78·5	2860
Female not insured persons ...	66·9	2439
Total male members	41·3	943
Total female members ...	44·3	1170

From the above it is observed that the amount of sickness, generally speaking, is greater in women than in men, but the sickness is less than among teachers.

Equally interesting data are obtained when a comparison is made between the various age-periods, no distinction being drawn between compulsorily and voluntarily insured persons.

Ages	Per 100 persons, cases of sickness		Days of sickness per individual	
	Male	Female	Male	Female
Under 15 years	38·0	29·0	5·9	5·5
15—20 years	37·6	36·4	6·3	8·0
20—25 ,,	36·3	42·1	6·9	10·4
25—35 ,,	38·0	50·2	8·0	14·2
35—45 ,,	44·3	55·3	11·0	16·7
45—55 ,,	51·7	54·3	14·9	16·9
55—65 ,,	60·2	54·9	21·2	19·6
65—75 ,,	75·7	66·6	33·2	27·4

The greater sick rate of females extends from puberty through the reproductive period of a woman's life. After the age of 55 women show a lower sick rate than men. Funk obtained statistics from the town of Bremen for 1901–1910 with the object of ascertaining how far the mortality of women was affected by social position and he found the following as the female mortality in percentages according to the three different classes:

At the age of	Well-to-do class of people	Middle class	Poor	Average
15—30... ...	42	74	113	60
30—60... ...	54	66	65	60
60 and upwards	88	95	97	92

Between the ages of 15 and 30 poor women have in Bremen only one-third of the chances of life of the well-to-do. Statistics obtained by Sörensen for Copenhagen do not quite confirm Funk's findings. Compared with these Westergard gives the following figures as applicable to Fuenen in Sweden:

At the age of	Wives and daughters of large farmers	Wives and daughters of middle class farmers	Female field workers
15—20 ...	115	152	170
20—25 ...	133	107	107
25—35 ...	153	153	156
35—45 ...	129	146	154
45—55 ...	106	99	89
55—65 ...	100	99	89
65—75 ...	98	102	92
75—85 ...	92	90	79
Above 85 ...	89	92	86

It is hardly possible to draw absolute conclusions from the preceding tables. On the whole the results are favourable especially, during the active part of a woman's life, to the well-to-do classes. A comparison of male and female mortality does not give a final answer to the influence of social position upon mortality. The diseases which fall more heavily upon the poorer working classes than the well-to-do are tuberculosis, affections of the respiratory and circulatory organs, diseases of the nervous system and digestive organs, and to these may be added cancer. Anæmia and chlorosis are maladies most noticeable in the early years of womanhood from 15–20, and to the causation of which long continued sitting when at work, or its opposite much standing, deprivation of fresh air and too short intervals for taking food contribute. The fact that, until recently in all countries, women when pregnant were allowed to continue at their employment in the factory and elsewhere almost to the end of term, was no doubt responsible for much of their subsequent ill-health, as were also the absence of home nursing during the lying-in period and the deficient or improper food supplied. Factory and other occupations keep attracting larger and larger numbers of women, and as motherhood is regarded as a disqualification for work restriction of family has become a noticeable feature of social life.

BIBLIOGRAPHY

"Krankheit und Soziale Lage." Article by Dr Wilhelm Weinberg, Stuttgart.

CHAPTER VII

DUSTY OCCUPATIONS

DUST AND WHAT IT IS COMPOSED OF. LEAD AND ITS COMPOUNDS. LEAD POISONING. COAL MINING. GOLD MINING AND MINERS' PHTHISIS

The greatest enemy of a worker in any trade is dust. If we could get rid of dust and have our people working in a clear and, comparatively speaking, dustless atmosphere we would hear less of occupational diseases. The dust given off in any particular trade may be of an organic nature like the fine fluff from cotton, or be inorganic like the particles of stone evolved in steel grinding, or particles of lead arising in the manufacture and handling of white lead. Some kinds of dust are soluble in the juices of the animal body, others are insoluble. The dust given off during work may be inhaled during respiration or it may become caught in the saliva of the mouth and be swallowed. Some dusts irritate the mucous membranes and induce coughing and running at the eyes, others owing to their chemical constitution, e.g. chrome salts and arsenical compounds, act as destructive agents and cause ulceration, or they cause general poisoning. The dust given off in mines during rock drilling is, when inhaled, a source of pulmonary diseases to which as a group the term *pneumoconioses* is applied. The pulmonary disease met with in gold miners is the result of breathing a dust-ladened atmosphere, but Calmette of Lille and his followers are of the opinion that the dust which creates the disease of the lungs does not reach these organs by inhalation but is swallowed, penetrates the intestinal mucous membrane, reaches the lymphatics and finally comes by the blood stream to the lungs. Calmette is also of the opinion that the tubercle bacillus which is the cause of tuberculosis reaches the lung not by the respiratory passage, but by the gastro-intestinal canal.

We must remember however that dust is something more than merely particles of an organic or inorganic nature. Usually the particles of dust which rise with the air are surrounded by a watery envelope and clinging to this moist covering there may be micro-organisms. An outbreak of tetanus among the jute workers of Dundee a few years ago was shown to be due to the spores of tetanus attached to the particles of dust which rose into the air of the factory and were inhaled by the workers. To the atmosphere in which a man is working there is added from his own body through the expired air and insensible perspiration, an amount of water equal to 15 to 20 grammes per hour. The moisture which encircles the particles of dust makes those particles not only carriers of micro-organisms, but also the medium wherein micro-organisms may multiply, so that two kinds of germs may be present in the air, those given off for example by a patient who is the subject of an infectious disease and those which, multiplying in the atmosphere, acquire characters of their own. Persons working in a dusty atmosphere may therefore become the subjects of an infectious

disease like tuberculosis, they may develop maladies of a
chronic nature like pulmonary consumption or general poisoning
as in plumbism. Some dusts are of an explosive nature as
witness the firing of flour mills and sugar factories. Until two
decades ago, the cotton operatives in Lancashire suffered in
larger proportion from pulmonary consumption than persons
engaged in other occupations in the same districts. The
morbidity rate has gradually been reduced by better ventilation
of the factories and by increasing the humidity of the air in
the work rooms.

Dr Edgar L. Collis, H.M. Medical Inspector of Factories,
and whose work in connection with dust diseases is well
known, draws attention to the fact that cotton operatives
suffer from attacks of difficulty of breathing which are different
in causation and character from ordinary spasmodic asthma.
Typical dust-asthma which he had seen among cotton strippers
is associated with a physical configuration of the chest and a
form of breathing entirely different from that observed among
operatives who experience a heavy mortality from dust phthisis.
Cotton strippers are exposed in the first processes of cotton
spinning to dust arising from cotton husk and debris which is
thrown in a fine cloud into the air when the cylinders of cotton
carding-machines are brushed out or "stripped." The coarser
grades of cotton give the greater amount of dust. From Surat
and American cotton more dust arises than from the finer
grade cotton which comes from Egypt. As each spinning mill
deals only with material of special grades the effect of the
different amounts of dust can be studied at different mills.
Thus Collis found among men working on coarse grades of
cotton that 91 per cent. were more or less affected, on medium
grades 72 per cent. and on fine grades 62 per cent. He also
found that cotton weavers suffer from an acute form of
spasmodic cough with asthmatic symptoms attributed by him
to inhalations of a special mildew which from time to time
settles on the cotton thread.

As an illustration of the irritating effects of industrial dust
mention may also be made of the running at the nose, fits of
sneezing, coughing, dryness of throat and smarting of the eyes

which are observed in men who are employed in sawing certain kinds of box-wood, e.g. *macaibo*. In the manufacture of shuttles for weaving purposes Professor Harvey Gibson of Liverpool found that the men who made the shuttles from West African box-wood suffered from headache, running at the nose, excessive secretion of tears and asthma. Professor Dixon of Cambridge obtained from the wood an alkaloid which when tested experimentally was found to be a cardiac depressant and to paralyse the nerve endings in muscle. From certain kinds of African box-wood which I submitted to Messrs Brady and Martin, chemists, Newcastle-upon-Tyne, certain alkaloids and glucosides were extracted for me but beyond inducing dilatation of the pupil they produced no constitutional disturbance.

The local irritating effects of soot are well known. It is the cause of cancer of the skin in chimney sweeps and is the cause of sores on the hands and forearms of gardeners who use it for sprinkling plants. These sores may or may not be due to arsenic contained in the soot.

Space will only allow of me dealing with two or three dusty trades. In one class the effects of the dust are local and general, in other trades the effects are general or constitutional. In the case of men who handle or mix arsenical pigments, Scheele's green for example, if proper precautions are not taken, the arsenical dust gets under the finger nails and also under any loose clothing. The dust produces ulceration of the skin so that portions of a finger have been known to become eaten away. In addition, owing to the men breathing the dust, the particles of arsenic settle down upon the nasal mucous membrane and in course of time cause perforation of the septum. The round opening which varies in size from a split pea to nearly a three-penny piece can be seen and felt. Although the opening which leads to a communication being established between the two nasal passages is the result of a destructive process it is astonishing how little inconvenience or pain is caused by the perforation. These openings never heal. In addition to perforation of the nasal septum and to ulceration of the skin in the flexures of the body and on the genitalia, there may be constitutional symptoms the result of the dust having been swallowed. The men suffer from headache and they lose weight and in some instances there occurs a loss of power in the lower extremities below the knee owing to neuritis. The above is an illustration of work in a dusty atmosphere causing both local and general symptoms.

Persons employed in the manufacture of white lead or the handling of it, suffer from a general form of poisoning to which the term plumbism, saturnism or lead poisoning is applied. White lead (carbonate) is largely used as a paint for buildings and for ships so that both the persons who make it and those who use it may suffer in their health. White lead is made by acting upon strips of metallic lead with the vapour given off from diluted acetic acid in chambers strewn with the disused bark obtained from a tanner's vat and closed in so that the heat which develops during the fermentation of the tan causes evaporation of the acetic acid. This vapour acts upon the metallic lead and converts it into the soluble acetate but the carbonic acid which is evolved from the tan overrides this action and converts the acetate into the carbonate. This process known in the trade as the *Dutch method* is slow: it requires 10–11 weeks for corrosion to take place. In what is known as the *chamber process* acetic acid is placed in jars on the floor of a special chamber, strips of metallic lead are hung over frames and carbonic acid gas from burning coke is carried into the chamber which is hermetically closed and its temperature gradually raised. A similar interaction takes place here between the acids and the metals as in the Dutch process but conversion is quickened by a few weeks.

By whichever method the lead has become converted into the carbonate, emptying of the chambers and stripping of the white lead are attended by the raising of considerable quantities of dust. Some of the men who are engaged in this work suffer from acute pain in the abdomen, known as lead colic; they also complain of severe headache and they may vomit. Some men are readily affected. There is an individual as well as a sexual idiosyncrasy to lead. Young persons and especially young females are especially prone to plumbism. The

abdominal pains complained of are frequently severe. It is
not uncommon to see the victims of lead colic writhe in agony,
and only obtain relief by pressing the abdomen, by the
application of external warmth or by the administration of
morphia. Occasionally abdominal pain is of the particular
type in which pressure cannot be borne. Accompanying the
pain there is usually obstinate constipation but enforced action
of the bowels by means of aperients although called for is
not always followed by relief of the abdominal pain. Instead
of colic, workers in lead may develop what is known as "wrist-
drop" or paralysis of the hands from the wrists downwards.
Usually both hands are affected, they hang helplessly by the
side of the body. The wrists cannot be extended nor can the
fingers. This form of paralysis which is typical of lead
poisoning is extremely unfitting to the individual. If the
paralysis is extreme the patient can neither dress nor feed
himself. Recovery too is slow. It may take months for the
paralysis to disappear.

While abdominal pain and paralysis of hands are of common
occurrence in plumbism there has generally been observed before
the development of these symptoms a degree of pallor of the
face. On enquiry too it is elicited that the workman has not
been taking his food well, that he has experienced an unpleasant
taste in the mouth and on separating his lips there can be seen
a blue line on the gums close to the teeth. Where the teeth
have fallen out or been removed there is no blue line. This
line known as the Burtonian may be transitory or fairly
permanent. If it cannot be washed away by rinsing the mouth
with warm water or gentle friction with a tooth brush, it is
of importance from a diagnostic point of view. In a white
lead worker the transitory blue line is due to the deposition
of white lead dust on the gum but the more permanent line is
due to particles of lead deposited in the deeper tissues of the
gum. These particles have been taken up by the living cells
and have become converted into black sulphide of lead through
the operation of sulphur compounds present in the mouth.
The blue line is not a sign that the individual is at the time of
its detection suffering from lead poisoning, it means that he

has lead in his system and that at any time symptoms of plumbism may arise.

Where therefore a man or woman gives a history of having worked in lead, or even without such a history, the presence of anæmia, a blue line on the gums, the history of abdominal pain, severe headache, or loss of power of the wrists, the diagnosis of lead poisoning may be made with certainty. It is in cases where there is no history of colic, no paralysis and no blue line on the gums that a difficulty arises in regard to diagnosis.

Persons who are absorbing lead into their system only escape having plumbism so long as they keep eliminating the metal from their body. The two main channels by which lead is thrown out of the body are the kidneys and the intestinal canal. In the urine and fæces of a person who is storing up lead in his tissues, or is passing lead through his body, the metal may be found in the urine. The presence of lead in the urine, like the blue line on the gums, although not a sign that the individual is at the time suffering from lead poisoning, is yet of great importance from a diagnostic point of view, for should by the merest chance elimination be checked through disorder of the emunctory organs, symptoms of lead poisoning would quickly arise. Men and women, in whose urine lead is detected on chemical analysis, resemble in some respects those persons in whose urine typhoid bacilli are found and yet who remain free from signs of the disease. A woman who has thus absorbed the metal and is known as a "lead carrier" may not present any signs of lead poisoning and yet she is capable of affecting her infant should she become pregnant.

Men too can continue to work in lead for years without showing signs of plumbism, but all the while there may be silently developing changes in the body, especially the kidneys, so that albumen will sooner or later be found in the urine, the arteries thickened and the heart hypertrophied. When these develop there is the possibility of rupture of a cerebral blood vessel taking place, so that cerebral hæmorrhage is thus the final link in a chain of morbid events, the first link of which was forged by the altered metabolism of the body consequent upon the absorption of lead.

Women are more readily affected by lead than men. They suffer too from the worst types of it. Their sexual life is readily deranged by the metal. Menstruation becomes excessive and women if pregnant tend to miscarry. A large percentage of pregnant lead workers fails to reach term. Should they succeed the infants are either stillborn or they die in convulsions shortly after birth. It was knowledge of the great loss of infantile life, and of the severity of plumbism in women, which forced me to suggest to the Home Office the abolition of female labour in the dangerous processes of white lead factories. The good which has followed this restriction, the infantile life saved and the suffering prevented have more than been a compensation for the inconveniences caused to the trade and the temporary increased cost of production. It has made the industry healthier. As already stated females suffer from the worst forms of lead poisoning. They experience severe headache, and without having colic or wrist-drop they may pass without warning into convulsions in which they die, or if they recover from these their eyesight is temporarily or permanently lost.

The treatment of industrial lead poisoning is preventive and curative. Cases of plumbism arising from occupation must be reported by medical practitioners to the Factory Department of the Home Office. For each notification a fee of half a crown is allowed. By early notification of such cases industrial plumbism has frequently been checked so to speak in the bud. Defective plant in lead factories has been thus early detected and remedied. Owing to the present regulations enforced by the factory department of the Home Office, the amount of lead poisoning in this country has considerably declined during the last quarter of a century. Plumbism occurs in persons following diverse occupations. In addition to being met with in lead workers the malady occurs in potters, especially in persons employed in the dipping shop since the glaze usually contains lead: it is met with too in house and ship painters, in colour grinders and occasionally in factories where certain kinds of stained wool are manipulated. It is because lead is made use of in upwards of 110 industries that the metal is so important from a commercial, industrial and medical point of view. Periodical medical examination of the workers with power of suspension, restriction of female labour in all dangerous processes, greater attention to the personal hygiene of the employees and improved methods of working have removed from the manufacture of white and red lead many of the dangers to health incidental to the trade.

As regards curative measures, the treatment for colic must be conducted on general lines. Application of warmth to the abdomen, the administration of castor oil if there is no vomiting, or a draught of sulphate of magnesia with carminatives will probably give relief. Should these fail a warm bath may be tried, or morphia given hypodermically. If there is vomiting this may be relieved by an effervescing mixture of soda and bismuth with or without tinct. belladonna or morphia. For the dull aching pain which continues and which does not disappear after the action of aperients, I find half to one grain doses of mono-sulphite of soda most useful. Dr G. A. Stephens of Swansea finds permanganate of calcium in $\frac{1}{4}$ grain doses thrice daily helpful. Iodide of potassium and magnesium sulphate are recommended by some physicians, but these should be administered with care.

Several months ago Mr T. M. Clague of Newcastle-upon-Tyne and myself introduced what is known as the "double electrical bath treatment of plumbism." Under its influence lead stored up in the body we found was eliminated. We found electricity to be not only a curative but a preventive agent as well. The apparatus which is of an extremely simple nature has been fitted up in several white lead factories. From some factories encouraging accounts come of the result of the treatment: from others the accounts are less encouraging. In our own hands good results have been obtained. The duration of colic was, in Dr Patterson's patients in Philadelphia, U.S.A., very much shortened, so too was the duration of the paralysis, and the so-called "chronic rheumatic" and ill defined pains in the joints and limbs complained of by the older workers. The bath is of the simplest character—it is a foot bath and an arm bath only. Into the foot bath containing warm water with a little salt the positive pole of an electric battery is dropped, and into the arm and hand bath the negative pole. When the patient's arms and feet are immersed therein the electrical current traverses the body. Both on the poles and in the water of the bath, especially the negative, lead has been found. The double electrical bath is well worthy of a trial. It is not maintained that it can accomplish everything in the treatment of plumbism or that during its use other methods of treatment are to be disregarded. For the double wrist-drop and the loss of muscle substance which accompanies the paralysis local electricity other than that already described may be tried, also the administration of tincture of Nux Vomica by the mouth or Liq. Strychniæ hypodermically.

When the kidneys have become affected and there is anæmia, also signs of general deterioration of the body, the treatment must be that of symptoms, due attention being paid to the heightened blood pressure which is such a frequent accompaniment of the condition.

After death traces of lead are frequently found in the liver, kidneys, muscles and brain.

Inorganic Dust

Coal mining, gold mining and steel grinding

Half a century ago and less, the mortality of coal miners in this country from pulmonary consumption was greater than it is to-day. When a coal miner died in those days and his chest was opened the lungs were found to be perfectly black: portions of them were solid, while other portions were excavated. When the organs were squeezed there escaped a black ink-like fluid. During life, affected miners kept bringing up large quantities of "black spit": they declined in health, lost flesh and as the course of their illness resembled that observed in ordinary pulmonary consumption they were said to be the victims of "coal miners' phthisis" or to use the medical term "anthracosis." The compulsory use of the double shaft in coal mines, the pumping in of air through the main ways and the means adopted underground for diverting the ingoing air into proper channels and making it circulate towards the up-shaft have so improved the atmosphere of coal mines and the working conditions therein that the calling of the miner is no longer regarded as the unhealthy occupation it was half a century ago. Over-ventilation of coal mines however by drying the air too much and whisking through the passages the very fine dust which has settled down on the ledges of the rock and the beams of wood may of itself create dangers of quite another kind.

The comparative freedom of the coal miner to-day from phthisis is admittedly the result of the improved conditions under which he works. Although a coal miner's lung is usually quite black it seldom gives rise to consumption, unless the coal which is being hewed contains a considerable quantity of stone and grit. The carbon particles of soft coal do little damage to the lungs. It is otherwise with the gold miner of the Rand. It is now 13–14 years since I drew the attention of the medical profession and the gold mining fraternity to the large numbers of comparatively speaking young men who were dying from lung disease as a result of working in the gold mines of the Transvaal. Healthy men who had gone from the north of England to take up gold mining in South Africa returned six years or so afterwards with their purse well filled, but they themselves ruined in health and likely to die a few months afterwards from *silicosis* or *gold miners' phthisis*. This is a dust disease of the lungs. Gold miners' phthisis is the greatest evil the mining magnates of South Africa have to fight. The mines are deep. Ventilation is bad and the temperature is high. Some of the conditions under which the work was carried on have been improved. The rock is pierced by drills driven mostly by compressed air. These rock drills when in operation raise thick clouds of fine dust if water is not at the same time sprayed upon the rock. It is this fine dust which when inhaled sets up the structural changes in the lungs whereby they cease to be sponge-like organs capable of absorbing and retaining air and become converted into solid organs, unfitted for the purposes of aeration of the blood.

Another circumstance which favours the development of the disease is that after firing the cartridges of dynamite and bringing down the rock the miners enter too soon into the particular place where they were working, that is before the fumes of the explosive have passed away and the dust has had time to settle. When once the dust has taken a firm hold upon the lungs of the miners who have inhaled it and those structural changes are begun which ultimately lead to the soft spongy tissue of the lungs becoming converted into a hard fibrous material, the men begin to decline in health, they suffer from recurrent colds on the chest, they become short of breath and are unable, when the disease is well developed, to walk a few paces without panting. In a few instances where the men have been the subjects of the minor forms of the disease and have continued to follow their occupation some of them have died suddenly in the mine from heart failure. In the majority of cases the men become the subjects of cough. They become emaciated, they lose strength and are obliged to give up the work. It is but few rock drillers who survive more than six or seven years spent in this occupation. Gold miners' phthisis is less prevalent than it was two decades ago.

The publication of my paper in the *Lancet* was the cause of the South African Government appointing a commission to enquire into the subject. The findings of the commission confirmed the statements I had made so that steps were ultimately taken to improve the conditions under which mining operations were carried out on the Rand. I have always maintained that the difference between gold miners' phthisis and ordinary pulmonary consumption is that the former at its inception is a purely dust disease and only later on becomes tuberculous by the bacillus of Koch becoming engrafted upon it. Get rid of the dust in the mine therefore and much of the phthisis will disappear. Men whose bronchial tubes are the seat of recurrent catarrh and whose lungs have become irritated by dust are, if the fibrosis is not too well developed, more liable to be injuriously affected by the tubercle bacillus than those whose lungs are healthy. Rock drillers who are the subjects of phthisis receive compensation from their employer. If the disease is well developed the men are not allowed to continue at their occupation. They receive compensation to the extent of £8 per month for one year and are temporarily dismissed if not seriously ill.

The Miners' Phthisis Act was passed by the South African Government in 1912. For the eighteen months ending 31 January 1914 compensation amounting to £1,098,136 had been paid to miners or their dependants. With the exception of £100,000 which was gifted by the Government the whole of the money was paid by the Gold Mining Companies. It was equivalent to a tax of 7d. per ton of material milled during that period. As already stated if the miner's health is not seriously impaired he receives £8 per month for one year. Should the disease have developed to such an extent that fitness for work underground is permanently destroyed the Act allows £8 per month up to a maximum of £400 (in special cases to even a higher amount) and to the dependants of a miner who has died from miners' phthisis £400 in a single sum or *pro rata* in monthly instalments. On the Rand, miners' phthisis is regarded as an industrial disease. The death rate of miners consequent upon affections of the pulmonary organs is six times as great as that of the remaining population of the Transvaal.

It is only those patients whose disease is detected early and who are sent away into other employment, preferably of an open air type, who can regain their health, for once the malady has become well developed and the fibrosis commences to penetrate the lungs, the tendency is for the disease to become progressive and for the patient to die at a comparatively early age. Simultaneous water spraying and rock drilling have reduced the prevalence of miners' phthisis. If a gold miner who is the subject of pneumoconiosis becomes tuberculous and is allowed to follow his occupation there is the risk of his fellow workmen becoming infected. Better ventilation, shorter shifts, water spraying and greater delay in entering the particular

part of the mine after the firing of explosives will do much to
still further improve the conditions of deep mining in the
Transvaal.

As already stated the lungs of the gold miner become
transformed into a mass of hard tissue in which are imbedded
particles of the rock which have been inhaled in the form of
fine dust. These impart to the lungs on being cut by the knife
a gritty feeling and explain their stony hardness. A similar
condition of the lungs is found in men who work in other dusty
occupations, e.g. ganister mining and steel grinding. The
Sheffield trades are notorious for the large amount of pulmonary
disease in those who follow them. What has been said of the
gold miner applies equally well to the dry steel grinder. Stone
masons and workers in potteries also suffer from a similar
affection of the lungs. The so-called "potter's rot" frequently
commences as a bronchial catarrh whereby the ciliated epithelium which lines the windpipe and bronchi becomes removed.
The ciliated epithelium arrests the dust which has been inhaled
and prevents it reaching the lungs. The loss of this protective
barrier lays the workman open to his lungs becoming more
readily invaded by dust.

BIBLIOGRAPHY

Collis, Edgar L. Milroy Lectures delivered at Royal College of
    Physicians, London, 1915.
Oliver, Thomas. *Diseases of Occupation*. Messrs Methuen and Co.,
    London.
Oliver, Thomas. *Lead Poisoning*. H. K. Lewis and Co., London.
Oliver, Thomas. "Gold Miners' Phthisis." *Lancet*, June 14, 1902.
Reports of the Transvaal Chamber of Mines, 1913 on.
Cobbett, L. *The Spread of Tuberculosis*. (Cambridge Public Health
    Series.)

CHAPTER VIII

GASES

CARBON DIOXIDE.   CARBON MONOXIDE.   SULPHURETTED
HYDROGEN.   FERRO-SILICON.   NICKEL CARBONYL.   CARBON
BISULPHIDE

Carbonic Acid: Carbon Dioxide

Carbonic acid (CO_2) is when compared with carbon monoxide
(CO) and sulphuretted hydrogen (H_2S) a feeble poison. It is
the gas which is normally formed in the living body and is
eliminated in our breath during expiration. It is present in
the atmosphere to the extent of ·04 per cent. When the
percentage of carbonic acid is increased in the air we breathe,
as occurs occasionally in close, ill-ventilated and artificially
lighted work rooms, it causes headache, dizziness, a sense of
tiredness and a feeling of unfitness for work. Three per cent.
causes difficulty of breathing, 6 per cent. palpitation and
headache and 10 per cent. induces unconsciousness. One of
the early effects of the presence of an excess of carbon dioxide
in the blood is quickened breathing. If the heart beats more
quickly this is only momentary for soon the beats become
slower, the face becomes cyanosed, the extremities cold and
death may supervene without convulsions. It is thus that
persons die who are the subjects of chronic heart disease
attended by gradual cardiac failure. They are the victims of
slow poisoning by carbon dioxide. For much that we know of
the harmful effects of carbonic acid when inhaled in excess we
are indebted to Paul Bert who showed that if the air which is
breathed is not renewed it becomes harmful: the tension of the
oxygen in the atmosphere falls until it is insufficient for the
needs of respiration and there occurs anoxæmia followed by
asphyxia. In ordinary respiration we not only take into the
lungs oxygen to vitalize the tissues but in expiration we exhale

carbon dioxide. Anything therefore which hinders the elimination of carbon dioxide becomes a source of harmfulness. Carbonic acid gas is poisonous alike to the muscular and nervous tissues. Experiments have shown that it paralyses the muscle fibre of the heart.

During the fermentation of beer, large volumes of an almost pure carbon dioxide are evolved from the vats. The malthouse of a brewery is permeated with the gas so that means are usually taken to have the air renewed before men enter. Imprudence in this matter has been followed by death. During fermentation of grape juice and the cleaning out of wine vats men have succumbed to the influence of carbon dioxide. This is the gas which is given off from kilns during the burning of lime.

Elsewhere in this book attention is directed to the ventilation of factories and the requirements of the factory department of the Home Office in regard thereto. It is a requirement that 250 cubic feet of atmospheric air shall be provided for each individual during working hours and 400 if the work is carried on beyond 10 hours per day. Usually carbonic acid poisons slowly and reduces the vital resistance of the individual gradually, but in one case which I saw death came with startling and unexpected rapidity. The case was that of the captain of a Life Saving Brigade who when wearing a Proto-Fleuss helmet and apparatus had penetrated a considerable distance into the disused drift of an abandoned coal mine. After death the valve of the apparatus which supplies the oxygen was found to have been turned the wrong way. A party entered the drift but the captain leaving his comrades at a particular place travelled further into the drift. He clambered over two "falls." His lamp went out and a canary which he was carrying was seen on his return to be alive but not brisk. The man himself was observed to be in distress: his breathing was laboured and he made signs to his comrades of an enquiring nature as to whether his "dress" was all right. The gauge of the apparatus showed that he had still 15 minutes of oxygen supply left, that is 15 atmospheres (one atmosphere is equivalent to one minute of time). He commenced to run towards the mouth of the drift but he had only run a few yards when he fell down dead. When examined, respiration had ceased and the heart had stopped beating. I was present at the autopsy. The signs were those of asphyxia such as is caused by excess of carbon dioxide, viz. dilated right heart, left side of heart empty and flaccid, the lungs, liver and abdominal viscera deeply congested, so too the vessels of the brain.

The point I wish to emphasize is the sudden death of a healthy young man who was accustomed to, and in almost daily training for, life saving work and who therefore was familiar with the dangers incidental to it. There had taken place a slowly produced asphyxia from deprivation of oxygen: carbonic acid gas had slowly accumulated in the blood. Of the effects of the gas slowly accumulating the individual had evidently been aware, hence the question as to whether his "dress" was all right. Almost immediately after asking it he fell down dead. Such suddenness of death in carbon dioxide poisoning is quite unusual.

Carbon Monoxide

This gas is present to the extent of 7–10 per cent. in ordinary illuminating gas. It is the source of the blue flame which is seen in grates when a coal fire is burning brightly. It is the gas given off from coke ovens and which has been the cause of death to many tramps invited to the ovens on a winter's night and allured by their warmth to sleep. Carbon monoxide is a colourless gas and inodorous. It therefore poisons insidiously. When inhaled the gas enters into an extremely stable combination with the red-colouring matter or hæmoglobin of the red corpuscles of the blood so that they cease to take up oxygen from the atmospheric air and as a consequence the individual dies asphyxiated. A very small percentage of carbon monoxide gas is dangerous. Unpleasant sensations such as headache and a feeling as if the limbs could not give support are experienced when there is such a small quantity as 0·1 per cent. present in the air. When the amount rises to 0·4 per cent. it is dangerous.

Carbon monoxide is the gas given off from blast furnaces

when these are being charged or tapped. Blast furnace gas frequently contains as much as 25 to 40 per cent. of CO. It is this gas which is frequently present in coal mines after an explosion and which makes descent into such a mine in order to attempt rescue work without the men wearing helmets so dangerous. The effects of carbon monoxide may be acute or chronic. In the acute forms of poisoning the victims are suddenly overpowered and rendered unconscious. In some of those who have recovered I have been struck by the presence of nystagmus, a peculiar oscillatory movement of the eyeballs, which renders vision imperfect and creates a feeling of dizziness. Speech too is frequently deranged and the power of walking impaired. Occasionally mental effects are produced not unlike those met with in aggravated hysteria and in the early stages of general paralysis.

It is the carbon monoxide present in illuminating gas which causes it to be dangerous when breathed. Water gas, produced by passing steam over red hot coke, is occasionally added to coal gas to improve its illuminating properties. Water gas sometimes contains as much as 30 per cent. of carbon monoxide. As water gas has not the disagreeable odour of ordinary coal gas it may escape into a living room without being detected or even suspected until some persons are overcome by it. The Home Office has therefore recommended that water gas should be scented. The amount of carbon monoxide contained in water gas should not exceed 14 per cent.

Professor Glaister of Glasgow and Dr Dale Logan of Newmains have made valuable literary contributions to the subject of carbon monoxide poisoning. Dr J. S. Haldane's work on mine gases is deservedly well known and appreciated. Haldane has shown the length of time that is required for dangerous symptoms to appear in men when, unprotected, they are exposed to varying percentages of carbon monoxide gas. His researches have an important bearing upon rescue work in mines. The harmful influence of carbon monoxide is enhanced if during exposure to it muscular exercise is being indulged in at the same time, probably because deeper inspirations are taking place or the pulse rate is quickened and therefore a larger area of the blood is exposed in a given time to the gas. In an atmosphere containing 0·1 per cent. of CO a man at rest can breathe the gas for 2½ hours before the blood becomes saturated with it to the extent of 50 per cent., but if he is walking about one-half of this time will suffice to bring about saturation. Men who undertake rescue work in an atmosphere containing 0·1 per cent. of CO begin to feel weak in their limbs and gradually lose power in them within one hour and even earlier if they are working hard. In 0·2 per cent. CO atmosphere men may be overcome in half an hour and in 0·3 per cent. atmosphere in twenty minutes. These limits of time are useful guides where men who are unprotected enter the gas zones in a mine. Men may reach a particular part in a mine and may be rescuing a comrade overpowered by gas when they themselves have not sufficient oxygen carrying hæmoglobin left in their blood to enable them to come back safely.

Men who have been overcome by CO gas and have recovered recite the same story so far as symptoms are concerned. Giddiness, ringing noises in the ears, fluttering of the heart and breathlessness on muscular effort are danger signals. When once these are experienced the men ought immediately to leave the particular place in the mine and make their way to where the air is purer. It is frequently when attempting to accomplish this that the limbs fail to carry their owner and he falls down in a state of stupor or of complete unconsciousness.

Where the poisoning has been of a less severe form the men subsequently complain of violent headache, they vomit, they have palpitation of the heart and there is muscular weakness or tremor. Glaister and Dale Logan describe one case of acute arterio-sclerosis as a sequel of carbon monoxide poisoning. The pulse was one of high tension: 240 mm. Hg. instead of the normal 130. Sudden death has been observed in carbon monoxide poisoning owing probably to the gas exercising a paralysing influence upon the nerves of the heart or upon the nerve centres in the medulla oblongata. In some of my own experiments I found minute hæmorrhages in the brain of animals who had died from acute CO poisoning.

After an explosion in a coal mine men are frequently found

lying in a state of complete unconsciousness. These men when brought to bank may yet be restored although a few of them may develop and succumb to pneumonia as a sequel of carbon monoxide toxæmia.

My attention has been directed to certain complaints as regards health by men employed at coke ovens where such bye-products as benzol, toluol and sulphate of ammonia are recovered. They complain of loss of appetite, derangement of the digestive organs and a sense of increasing weakness. We are not familiar with the effects of the inhalation of carbon monoxide in minute doses carried on over a long period. The men certainly become pale, almost greenish pale, in colour and their vital resistance is reduced. At the bye-product ovens the men are exposed to various gases, but probably the most deleterious of these is carbon monoxide. I have for several hours a day and for a period of many weeks exposed animals to an atmosphere containing o·25 per cent. of carbon monoxide with the result that with increased frequency of exposure to the gas, not only are the animals more quickly overcome by the carbon monoxide and rendered helpless by it but they lose weight. This may be regained. Instead of the blood becoming paler the number of red blood corpuscles increased by one to two millions and the amount of hæmoglobin or colouring matter rose in proportion.

Sulphuretted Hydrogen

This is an extremely poisonous gas. It is frequently present in the sewers of large towns especially when these subterranean channels have become blocked. Labourers who have entered these underground passages have occasionally died suddenly. Minute quantities of the gas o·2 to o·4 per cent. are dangerous. Sulphuretted hydrogen acts upon the respiratory nerve centres also upon the terminal endings of the pneumo-gastric nerves in the lungs. I have succeeded in restoring animals asphyxiated by sulphuretted hydrogen by means of the oxygen pulmometer, but to restore life the application must be made immediately death is supposed to have taken place.

Ferro-Silicon

Pig iron contains varying percentages of ferro-silicon. In ordinary pig iron there may be only 2 to 3 per cent. but in the softer forms there may be 15 per cent. During the last few years, owing to growing demands, high grade ferro-silicon has been prepared on a large scale. Where ferro-silicon is brought into contact with moisture, phosphuretted and arseniuretted hydrogen gases are evolved. These are powerful poisons. During the transport of ferro-silicon by sea especially in rough weather sailors on board of ship have died from the liberation of these gases consequent upon the cargo becoming moist.

Nickel Carbonyl

Nickel carbonyl is a poisonous liquid obtained from nickel copper oxide. It is extremely volatile. Nickel carbonyl is made in air-tight iron chambers but as the result of the vibration of the machinery leakages take place. Workmen have thus been suddenly and fatally overcome by the gas or they have died two or three days afterwards from acute congestion of the lungs. One of my laboratory animals after having breathed only a few drops of nickel carbonyl died 2 or 3 days afterwards and in its brain small hæmorrhages were found, also acute chromolytic changes in the nerve cells of the medulla oblongata. These minute hæmorrhages resemble those found in carbon monoxide poisoning. Medical opinion is still divided as to whether when a fatal termination has followed the inhalation of nickel carbonyl, death is due to the carbon monoxide contained in the carbonyl or is the result of the action of the nickel itself.

Bisulphide of Carbon

Bisulphide of carbon is obtained by passing sulphur vapour over red hot coal in cast iron retorts into which sulphur is introduced. When purified, bisulphide of carbon is a clear liquid with a disagreeable odour. It is used as a vulcanizing agent and as a solvent of india-rubber, also for the destruction of vermin. India-rubber is rendered more permanently elastic when combined with sulphur. Vulcanisation of rubber goods is effected with the aid of heat and pressure by means of such sulphur holding compounds as sulphide of barium and calcium, also by chloride of sulphur and in the cold by dipping the goods into a mixture of bisulphide of carbon and chloride of sulphur.

Now that the dangerous properties of bisulphide of carbon have become well known there have been during recent years in rubber factories fewer cases of poisoning than formerly. Paralysis has been known to follow inhalation of even such small quantities of the vapour as 1 mgm. per litre of air. I have seen neuritis with loss of power in the arms of rubber workers, also a peculiar series of brain symptoms such as are occasionally met with in acute insanity. Improved ventilation of work rooms, wider knowledge of the dangers of bisulphide of carbon and the enforcement of regulations have made the manufacture of india-rubber goods a less harmful industry than formerly.

Bisulphide of carbon produces, in young female workers, intoxication, in some respects not unlike that caused by alcohol: they stagger when walking and occasionally fall: on reaching home at the end of a day's work they frequently fall sound asleep before having tasted their supper. Sleep is heavy and unrefreshing. In the morning they awake with a splitting headache relieved by returning to the factory and again inhaling the vapour of the bisulphide. Sickness and vomiting are common symptoms. By repeated exposure to the vapour the nervous system becomes profoundly affected as evidenced by loss of muscular power, twitching and wasting of muscle substance, also by loss of eyesight. There is in many persons a stage of excitement attended by loquacity and when this passes away there is frequently mental depression accompanied by defective memory and impaired power of speech. Once developed, muscular tremors are slow to disappear. Most of the patients poisoned by bisulphide of carbon recover, but recovery is slow. Persons of a highly strung nature, with a leaning towards hysteria should not be allowed to work where bisulphide of carbon is used.   The work rooms should be well ventilated and naked lights owing to inflammability of the vapour must not be allowed.

On account of the poisonous properties of carbon bisulphide substitutes have been sought for it, such as benzine and carbon-tetrachloride, but these too have been found not to be free from danger.

BIBLIOGRAPHY

Glaister, Prof., and Dale Logan. *Gas Poisoning in Mining and other Industries.* Edinburgh, E. and S. Livingstone, 1914.

CHAPTER IX

THE CHEMICAL TRADES

Of all the sciences chemistry and electricity play the most important part in modern industry.   By the aid of chemistry artificial substitutes are replacing natural organic compounds. Man's wants are being met by the fertility of the chemical laboratory.   In medicine not less than in commerce is this the case.   The discovery of the aniline compounds and the increasing application of colloid chemistry have opened up fresh lines of research.   New processes keep replacing older methods of production.   It is when processes of manufacture pass from the experimental stage to production on a large scale that dangers to health and risk to life hitherto unsuspected are suddenly or slowly revealed.   In the recovery of material from bye-products lies one of the greatest achievements of modern chemistry.

Sulphur and Sulphur Miners

If the supply of sulphur were to fail, industrial chemistry would lose one of its most valuable assets.   Most of the sulphur made use of in Europe comes from Sicily.   Sulphur mining as carried on in Sicily is hard and degrading work.   The mines are hot and most of them are not ventilated in the proper sense of the word.   Sulphur is found in a comparatively pure state in the ore.   The men who get the ore by means of a pick are known as *picconieri*, while the boys who carry up a flight of stairs to the surface pieces of ore on their shoulders are called *carusi*.   The heat is so great that the men work in the mine without clothing.   I have visited the men in the sulphur mines of Sicily and can therefore bear testimony to the hard character of the work and its exhausting influence upon those who follow the employment.   The men can only work from 20 to 30 minutes at a time.   The muscular strain causes hypertrophy of the heart, the foul air induces anæmia, while inhalation of the sulphur dust and fume causes catarrh of the respiratory organs which Dr Alfonso Giordano of Lercara says frequently ends in a form of fibrosis of the lungs to which he has given the name of *theapneumoconiosis* the final termination of which is frequently pulmonary tuberculosis.

Another scourge of the sulphur miner in recent years has been *ankylostomiasis* or *miners' worm disease*.   The ankylostoma is a small worm-like parasite which when it reaches the upper part of the small intestine fastens itself by means of its hooklets to the mucous membrane of the alimentary canal and sucks the blood of its host, thereby inducing anæmia and at the same time a form of blood poisoning which render the miner unfit for work.   The presence of the ova and larvæ of the ankylostoma in the mines is an interesting fact when taken in conjunction with the bactericidal and parasiticidal properties of sulphur.

Until the last few years a Sicilian boy would enter the mine as a *caruso* or ore-carrier at an early age, 10–12 years or even earlier.   The age has recently been raised.   In hardly one of the mines, except a few of the largest, is there a lift.   The entrance into the mine is by a series of steps cut out of the rock.   In one mine which I visited there were 1000 steps up which men had to climb after a hard day's work.   Up similar but fewer steps in total darkness in another mine I found boys carrying large loads of sulphur ore on their shoulders.   The weights carried are too heavy.   The *carusi* emerge from the mouth of the mine panting, pale and with their heart beating at a much quickened rate.

As a consequence of the heavy weights which are carried and the impure air which is breathed, growth of the body becomes checked so that if a *caruso* continues to be an ore-carrier year after year he never attains to the stature of man but remains dwarfed both physically and mentally. His spine too becomes crooked so that in a sulphur mining district it is almost impossible for the Italian government to get conscripts for the army.

About 360,000 tons of sulphur are produced in Sicily annually. The mines give employment to 23,077 men and boys. Owing to competition from California and Louisiana the production of sulphur by Sicily has fallen lately. Many of the smaller mines have been closed. Owing to the fumes given off during the roasting of the sulphur, the country in the neighbourhood of the mines is barren.

Sulphuric Acid

In Great Britain sulphur dioxide is obtained by roasting pyrites in specially constructed furnaces or by burning brimstone. Sulphur dioxide is the basis of sulphuric acid. For the methods of manufacture of sulphuric acid text-books on chemistry must be consulted. What we have to deal with is the health of the workers. As regards that, it may be said that the men employed in sulphuric acid works do not suffer seriously in their health. In fact, of all chemical workers they suffer least. It is known however that a large percentage of them suffer from catarrhal affections of the respiratory organs owing to the irritating effects of the sulphur dioxide upon the mucous membrane of the bronchial tubes. Care has therefore to be exercised in cleaning out the Gay-Lussac towers of a chemical works that the men do not inhale the strong acid vapours, for workmen have succumbed a few hours after having been exposed to them. In sulphuric acid there are frequently impurities. One of the most dangerous of these is arsenic. Here it may be incidentally stated that serious symptoms follow inhalation of arseniuretted hydrogen. Of these hæmaturia and jaundice are the most pronounced.

Hydrochloric Acid

In the manufacture of soda by the Leblanc process the hydrochloric acid in Great Britain was formerly allowed to escape into the atmosphere, but it had a destructive influence upon vegetation, hence the barren condition of the surrounding country in close proximity to chemical works. The manufacture of soda by the Leblanc process consists primarily in producing sodium sulphate from common salt and sulphuric acid. Hydrochloric acid is then formed. The Alkali Acts require that the hydrochloric acid shall not escape but after being condensed shall be absorbed in water and for this product a ready market is found. Sodium sulphate and sodium sulphide are also produced. The teeth of the men who work in the hydrochloric acid department become eroded, and in the department where caustic soda is produced care has to be taken that the splashes of caustic soda do not fall upon the skin, otherwise these inflame the skin and cause it to ulcerate. During the pouring of lime into the hot soda lye, a second stage of the Leblanc process, the men have to watch that the contents of the vessel do not froth over, for severe injuries have been caused to the eyes by the lye spurting over.

Chlorine and Chloride of Lime

In the manufacture of these for bleaching purposes the workmen incur the risk of injuring their health by inhaling chlorine. According to Leymann 17·8 per cent. of the workmen employed in the chlorine department of chemical works suffer from diseases of the respiratory organs compared with 8·8 of persons employed in other processes. Many of the workmen suffer also from a rash on the skin called "Chlorine rash."

Nitric Acid

This is obtained from salt-petre or sodium nitrate. This is decomposed by means of sulphuric acid in cast iron retorts. The product in its crude state contains nitrous and nitric oxides. It is these which give to impure nitric acid its reddish colour. Burns are frequently met with among the workmen, so also are diseases of the respiratory organs to the extent of 11·8 per cent. The fumes of nitrous and nitric acid are poisonous. When a fire breaks out in a place where nitric acid is stored the men should not attempt to extinguish the flames unless they are wearing smoke helmets. In Newcastle-upon-Tyne nearly a quarter of a century ago a fire occurred in a chemical store where large quantities of the acid were kept. Two of the firemen who were unprotected died from acute hæmorrhagic engorgement of the lungs a few days after trying to extinguish the fire. They suffered severely in their chest.

Phosphorus

Since the British Government abolished the use of white phosphorus in the manufacture of lucifer matches, work in match factories has become a comparatively harmless occupation. Formerly the fume given off from white or yellow phosphorus was a frequent cause of necrosis of the jaw bone or "phossy jaw" in persons employed especially in the mixing, dipping and boxing departments of a factory. Most of the producing European countries joined the Berne Convention (1906) at which it was decided to replace white phosphorus by a harmless substitute, the sesquisulphide of phosphorus. Ordinary strike-anywhere matches as now in the British market are made from sesquisulphide of phosphorus. This possesses none of the harmful qualities of the white phosphorus. In addition to white phosphorus causing necrosis of the bone referred to it has occasionally caused death by septic inflammation of the membranes of the brain. The disease extends by contiguity of the upper jaw bone to the base of the skull and its living membranes. Death is sometimes due to septic broncho-pneumonia through the pus discharged from the decaying bone escaping into the mouth and being insufflated into the bronchi and lungs. All these maladies of lucifer match-makers are now things of the past. The only trouble sesquisulphide of phosphorus has given rise to is irritation of the skin but the dermatitis is of a comparatively mild nature and readily yields to treatment.

"Safety" matches, or as they are sometimes called "Swedish" matches, are made from amorphous red phosphorus and are comparatively speaking free from danger.

BIBLIOGRAPHY

Leyman quoted by Rambousek. *Industrial Poisoning.* London, Edward Arnold, 1913. Articles dealing with the Chemical Trades.
Dangerous Trades. Edited by Oliver. Articles on the Chemical Trades.

CHAPTER X

INJURIES CAUSED BY ELECTRICITY

The increasing use of electricity in industry and commerce has opened up new sources of danger to human life. More accurate knowledge of the generation and distribution of electrical currents has enabled man to some extent to obviate these, but the subtle fluid will for ever remain a source of danger to the unwary. The effects of powerful electrical currents are said to resemble those caused by lightning-stroke with this difference that while those of lightning-stroke are direct and are due to destruction or alteration of tissue, death in electric shock is more the result of effects produced upon the heart, respiration and nervous system. There is however not always this difference. Contact with a live wire may kill a person outright or there may be burns from which the wounded person recovers slowly, only to find that certain portions of the body are deeply scarred or that the patient has lost the ends of several of his fingers or toes. Deforming injuries are peculiar to electricity.

In speaking of electrical currents the terms *voltage* and *ampèrage* are used. By voltage is meant pressure, tension or electromotive force and by ampèrage intensity of the electrical current. Comparing an electrical current with a stream of water falling from a height, voltage or tension would be represented by the height of the waterfall and ampèrage by a cross section of the stream. It is difficult to say what pressure of electrical current comes within the limits of safety. There are two kinds of electrical currents, the *continuous* and *alternating*. As regards the harmful effects produced by electricity the current is usually spoken of in terms of voltage so that when a fatal accident has occurred the question is usually asked with what voltage was the wire charged at the time of the accident. It is impossible to say what voltages are safe for so much depends upon the conditions existing at the time of contact. One man was killed near Prague by coming into contact with a wire charged with a pressure of 95 volts, and yet electricians have touched wires carrying currents of such high pressure as 5000 volts without experiencing any ill effects. The tension of an electrical current is the first thing to be determined, but although a current of 100 to 150 volts is usually regarded as within the limits of safety, 200 to 300 volts as coming within the danger zone and all above 600 as likely to be fatal, no absolute reliance can be placed upon these statements. The British Board of Trade makes no distinction as to what are safe and unsafe voltages: 250 volts is the amount of current allowed to be supplied into private consumers' premises. In the United States of America criminals are put to death by means of powerful electric shocks. The voltage recommended for electrocution is 1500, but contact with such a high voltage has not in every instance caused immediate death.

The injuries inflicted by electricity depend upon voltage, the duration of the application and the moist or dry state of the skin of the victim at the time. Contact with both poles is more dangerous than with one alone, for thereby a more effective flow of current takes place. The skin offers resistance to the entrance of the current. The resistance is measured in terms of *ohms*. The hard, thickened and dry skin of a workman's hand offers greater resistance to the penetration of an electrical current than where the skin is soft, delicate and moist. Resistance to the current is offered at the points of entrance into and exit from the body. The point of exit from the body is usually, but not always, the feet.   Contact is most frequently unipolar, that is to say when a workman's hand or arm comes into contact with live metal, the current traverses the body and escapes to earth by the feet.   The condition of the boots of the workman at the time of the accident, also the state of the soil upon which he is standing, wet or dry, will determine whether the electrical current will prove fatal or not.

Alternating currents are almost twice as dangerous as *continuous*: they also differ somewhat in their action.   At high tension, continuous currents cause severe burning and considerable destruction of tissue.   Alternating currents cause less destruction.   The burns which follow contact with live metal are frequently very severe: they are irregular, deep, angry looking and are less painful than their appearance suggests: they are slow to heal probably in consequence of the finer termination of the nerve fibres having been destroyed. The effects produced by electrical currents upon the tissues are the result of the combined influence of thermal, chemical and electrolytical action, but especially of thermal and electrolytical.   The tissues are decomposed by the electrolytic action of the current.   The *ions* formed under these circumstances possess chemical affinities whereby new compounds are formed out of the decomposing tissues and these acting as toxins may be the cause of some of the pathological effects which follow electrical injuries.   The deeper tissues in the wound are charred and torn or they may have been removed altogether owing to the action of the intense internal heat.

It cannot be too strongly insisted upon that the effects produced upon the body by electrical currents depend largely upon the manner in which the currents enter and leave it. Good contact, a moist skin and damp boots may transform a current regarded simply as hazardous into one which may prove fatal, hence the necessity of men who work on electrified railways remembering that in wet weather there is greater danger.   One man whom I saw had accidentally placed his foot on a live rail.   He was immediately hurled forward. A signal-man close at hand who witnessed the accident immediately put on india-rubber gloves and hastening towards the injured person rescued him. The patient was unconscious and shortly afterwards developed convulsions. Unconsciousness lasted for several hours. The man's boots and clothing appeared to be normal, but on removing the boots his feet were found to be the seat of angry looking sores on the heels through which the bone was seen to be exposed. Recovery was slow. A youth aged 19 while standing on a concrete floor touched with his right hand a wire carrying 6000 volts alternating current. He received a shock. The palmar surface of the right hand was severely charred, also the plantar surfaces of the right toes. Subsequently there was considerable sloughing of the right hand with exposure of the flexor tendons necessitating amputation of the gangrenous fingers. Another patient whom I saw was a labourer aged 22 years who was admitted into the Royal Victoria Infirmary, Newcastle-upon-Tyne, under the care of my colleague Mr H. D. Angus, in a condition of unconsciousness, having received two hours previously a shock from a current of 20,000 volts. His shoulders, abdomen and limbs were in places charred. On the back of the head there was a large deep wound the floor of which was exposed occipital bone. He had a rapid pulse, 150 per minute: pupils were dilated: there were profuse perspiration, feeble heart's sounds and great restlessness notwithstanding the fact of unconsciousness. The patient died 7 hours after his admission into the infirmary. At the post-mortem examination there were found on removing the skull-cap acute inflammatory changes in the diploe of the occipital bone immediately underlying the superficial burn. On section of the brain a hæmorrhage about the size of a walnut was found in the occipital lobe corresponding to the site of the wound. There were numerous minute hæmorrhages in the surrounding white substance of the brain. Most of the internal organs were deeply congested: the bladder contained bloody urine free from sugar.

In order to ascertain how electrical shock causes death my colleague, Prof. Bolam, and I carried out a series of experiments upon animals. When death took place it was usually due to sudden arrest of the heart's action. Animals apparently killed by electricity could frequently be restored by artificial respiration.

Treatment is preventive and curative. All dangerous parts of machinery should be protected or marked off in *red* so as to indicate danger. Persons employed in generating stations and on electrified railways should have all the dangers explained to them and be instructed as to the means to be adopted for separating the individual from the live wire if he is still grasping it, also when having done so if the patient is not breathing to commence at once artificial respiration and to continue it, aided by relays of men, for three quarters of an hour or more.

Where an accident has occurred and the individual is still grasping a live wire, a fellow workman, especially if his hands are moist, must not take hold of the injured person as he himself might receive a fatal shock. India-rubber gloves should be worn. Where these are unobtainable *dry* rags should be wrapped round the hands of the rescuer. To cut a live wire strong scissors should be used on wooden handles.

The burns caused by electrical currents must be treated on ordinary surgical lines. If there is hæmorrhage the application of turpentine dressings will generally be found to arrest it.

CHAPTER XI

THE SKIN AND OCCUPATION

Grocers' itch, bakers' itch and sugar refiners' itch are familiar phrases and carry with them the suggestion of some connection of the disease with occupation. There is complaint of itching due to an eczematous rash on the back of the fingers and hands, the palmar surfaces remaining free. The commonest trade skin disease is eczema. About one-fourth of the cases of skin disease which medical men are called upon to treat are the result of occupation. Persons employed in certain dusty trades, e.g. colour mixing, occasionally suffer from ulcers of the skin due to the presence of arsenic in the pigments employed. Men who melt antimony frequently suffer from an irritating rash on the skin of chest and abdomen. Dyers have their hands stained with the particular dyes they are using. Callosities form on the skin when exposed to hard friction as in the handling of a pick.   It has always to be borne in mind when a workman consults a doctor for a skin eruption that the skin disease may have been there before the particular kind of work was undertaken and that what has happened has been simply an aggravation of the malady by the occupation.

Illustrations of the effects of intermittent pressure are seen in the thickened and tender finger ends of harpists, violinists and typists.   Housemaid's knee, an inflamed bursa in front of the knee cap or patella, is the result of excessive kneeling and friction.   A similar condition of the patellar bursa is met with in coal miners as the result of kneeling on the hard rock in the mine.   Among these men the affection is known as "beat knee." "Beat hand" is a similar affection due to the handling of, and friction caused by, the pick.

Allusion has been made in the preceding pages to the injuries to the skin caused by electricity.   The hands of persons who do X-ray work become thickened, unsightly and ultimately eroded or cracked.   Repeated and prolonged exposure to X-rays of high intensity was believed to be the cause of the cancerous sores which developed upon the forearm of Mr Thomas A. Edison's private secretary and which was also the cause of death in at least one radiographer who had been employed in the South African War.   Men employed in certain departments in chemical works develop ulcers on their skin as the result of exposure to acid fumes.   Alkalis have even a more destructive effect than acids.   Men exposed to the vapours from pitch and tar, also to splashes from oils obtained in the distillation of coal, develop warts.   These growths on the skin sometimes disappear and there are observed instead ulcers which tend to become malignant.

BIBLIOGRAPHY

White Prosser, R.   *Occupational Affections of the Skin.*   H. K. Lewis, London, 1915.

INDEX

Abdominal pains of workers in white lead manufacture, *see* lead colic
Accidents, causation of 7; occurrence of, in different occupations, 24 ff.
Acetic acid in manufacture of white lead 75
Acids, injuries caused by 103
Age and working capacity 36 f., 56 f.
Agriculture, percentage of persons employed in 1; the healthiest occupation 57
Air
 means of purifying 19 f.
 of factories, importance of 15
 stagnant, harmful effects of 15 f.
Air space in factories 51 f.
Alcohol
 raises sickness and mortality rates 66
 stimulation for work sought in 29 f.
Alkali Acts 96
Alkalis, injuries caused by 103
Ambulance instruction in factories 54
American cotton, dust from 73
Amorphous red phosphorus 98
Ampèrage of electrical currents 98 f.
Anæmia, causation of 71, 80, 94
Angus, H. D. 101
Aniline compounds 93
Animal life, injurious effects of chemical works on 9 f.
Ankylostoma in sulphur mines 94
Ankylostomiasis 94
Anoxæmia 85
Anthracosis 81
Anthrax 11
Anthrax bacilli 19
Antimony, rash of skin caused by 102
Anti-Sweating League 39 f.; Reports of 45
Apprenticeship, compulsory 4; legislation regarding 5
Arens on dust in air of workrooms 18
Arsenic, harmful effects of 58, 74, 102
Arseniuretted hydrogen gas 91, 95
Arterio-sclerosis 36, 89

Artificial flower making 40 ff.; much sickness connected with 42
Ascher, Dr Louis, of Königsberg 10, 15
Aspergilli 18
Aspergillus fumigatus 10, 19
Asphyxia 85, 87
Athens, number of slaves employed in 1 f.
Atmosphere, pollution of 11 ff.
Avenue St Cloud, examination of air from 13 f.

Bacillus aerogenes capsulatus in street dust 12
Bacillus anthracis 19
Bacillus coli in street dust 12
Bacteria in air 12 ff., 19 f.
Bakers' itch 102
Bath houses in factories 50 f.
Beat hand 103
Beat knee 103
Beer, fermentation of 86
Berne Convention of 1906 97
Bert, Paul, on effects of carbonic acid 85
Bethnal Green, sweated homes of 38 f.
Bisulphide of carbon, poisonous vapours from 91 ff.; effects of 92
Blast furnace gas 87 f.
Bolam, Professor, electrical experiments of 101
Box-wood, effects of dust from 74
Boys, occupations for 66 f.
Bremen, mortality statistics from 70
Breslau, small-pox epidemic in (1906) 43
Brick fields, conditions of labour in 44 f.
Brigue 50
Broken Hill mines, Australia 9
Bronchitis of feather sorters 43; of potters 58
Bryant, Col., Commissioner of Labour, New Jersey 47 f.
Building and construction, percentage of persons employed in 1

Rubber factories, cases of poisoning at 92
Rush of work tends to increase the mortality rate 56, 66
Rushing 26, 37
Russia, uncleansed feathers from 43

Sadler, Michael, introduction of the Ten Hours' Bill by 6
Safety matches 98
Sanitary Act of 1896 7
Sartory, A., and Langlais, M. 12 ff., 17 f., 22
Saturnism, causation of 75
Savage, Dr W. G. 15
Scheele's green 74
Schuler and Burckhard 35
Sesquisulphide of phosphorus 97
Sheffield trades and pulmonary disease 84
Shipyards, accidents in 23, 26; regulations regarding 54
Shredded Wheat Company's works 53
Shuttles, manufacture of 74
Sicily sulphur mines 93 ff.
Sickness, liability to, relation of, to age 37
Sickness rates
    a measure of the healthfulness of different industries 65
    circumstances which raise 66
    of males compared with that of females 35, 68 f.
Silicosis 81
Simplon tunnel 50
Skilled trades 66
Skin diseases caused by occupation 102 f.
Slag workers in Germany 11
Slaves, employment of, in industries 1 f.
Smith, George, of Coalville 44 f.
Social welfare of the workers 53
Soda, manufacture of 96
Sodium sulphate 96
Sodium sulphide 96
Sommerfeld, statistics of 21
Soot, effects of 74
Sörensen, mortality statistics of 70
South Africa
    Eastern Province of, feather sorters of the 43
    gold mines of 81 f.
South African War, radiographers of 103
Speeding up of machinery 26, 37
Spelter works, harmful effects of fumes from 9
Spinal deformity in brick makers 44; in Sicilian ore-carriers 95
Spittoons, use of, in factories 17

Staphylococcus pyogenes aureus 19 f.
Steam power, introduction of 2
Steel grinding, lung affections of workers in 84
Steinhaus, on methods of disinfecting feathers 43, 45
Stephens, Dr G. A., of Swansea 79
Sterilisator, electrical, for disinfecting air 20
Stettin, sickness rates from 68
Straker, William 57
Street dust 12
Streptococci 19
Sugar refiners' itch 102
Sulphur and sulphur miners 9, 93 ff.
Sulphur dioxide 95
Sulphuretted hydrogen 85, 90
Sulphuric acid 95
Sunday's rest 23 f., 29 f.
Surat cotton 73
Swansea 9
Sweated industries 38 ff.
Sweating, evils of 40
Swedish matches 98
Swiss International Exposition in Geneva (1896) 24
Switzerland, cotton mills of 35

Tarred roads and non-tarred roads, examination of air from 14
Tatham, Dr John 21 f., 55, 58 ff., 64
Taylor, Whateley Cooke 8
Teaching as an occupation for girls 68
Ten Hours' Bill of 1831 6
Tetanus among jute workers 72
Textile fabrics, percentage of persons employed in 1
Theapneumoconiosis 94
Tobacco smoke, the effect of, on dust in air 20
Trabonelli sulphur mine, Sicily 9
Trades Board Act of 1909 40
Traffic and dust 12 ff.
Transvaal Chamber of Mines, Reports of the 84
Transvaal gold mines 81 ff.
Trentham, U.S.A. 47 f.
Tubercle bacillus 12, 21
Tuberculosis
    and dusty occupations 17, 21, 58
    hastened by coal smoke 10
    percentages of, in certain trades in the State of Ohio 68
Tuberculosis aspergillaris 19

Ulcers of the skin caused by occupation 74, 102 f.
United Kingdom, percentages of persons engaged in different industries in 1

www.ingramcontent.com/pod-product-compliance
Ingram Content Group UK Ltd.
Pitfield, Milton Keynes, MK11 3LW, UK
UKHW040657180125
453697UK00010B/220